P9-DNX-113

For more than thirty years, pioneering nutritionist CARLTON FREDERICKS has been advocating diet as the most important factor in preventing disease. Author of the two-million-copy best seller *Low Blood Sugar and You,* he is now president of the International Academy of Preventive Medicine.

If you follow the diet advice in this sane and sensible book, you may reap dividends that will astonish you. The greatest reward, though, may be a negative one—what *doesn't* happen. The bowel cancer, appendicitis, diverticular diseases, hemorrhoids, and varicose veins that you *don't* get are very real, very tangible rewards!

CARLTON FREDERICKS'
HIGH-FIBER WAY TO TOTAL HEALTH
is an original POCKET BOOK edition.

Are there paperbound books you want but cannot find in your retail stores?

You can get any title in print in **POCKET BOOK** editions. Simply send retail price, local sales tax, if any, plus 25¢ (50¢ if you order two or more books) to cover mailing and handling costs to:

MAIL SERVICE DEPARTMENT
POCKET BOOKS • A Division of Simon & Schuster, Inc.
1 West 39th Street • New York, New York 10018

Please send check or money order. We cannot be responsible for cash.   *Catalogue sent free on request.*

Titles in this series are also available at discounts in quantity lots for Industrial or sales-promotional use. For details write our Special Projects Agency: The Benjamin Company, Inc., 485 Madison Avenue, New York, New York 10022.

Carlton Fredericks' High-Fiber Way to Total Health

by Carlton Fredericks

PUBLISHED BY POCKET BOOKS NEW YORK

CARLTON FREDERICKS' HIGH-FIBER
WAY TO TOTAL HEALTH

POCKET BOOK edition published January, 1976

4th printing.........................April, 1976

This original POCKET BOOK edition is printed from brand-new
plates made from newly set, clear, easy-to-read type.
POCKET BOOK editions are published by
POCKET BOOKS,
a division of Simon & Schuster, Inc.,
A GULF+WESTERN COMPANY
630 Fifth Avenue,
New York, N.Y. 10020.
Trademarks registered in the United States
and other countries.

ISBN: 0-671-80269-0.
Copyright, ©, 1976, by Carlton Fredericks. All rights reserved.
Printed in the U.S.A.

I dedicate this book to our youngest daughter, Rhonda, and our younger son, Spencer, in delighted appreciation of their loving tolerance for their father, their inexhaustible warmth, and their everyday romance with life

Contents

safe for some, a peril to others • How heredity influences enzyme chemistry

CONTENTS

9

CONTENTS

CONTENTS

A Personal Note

"Greetings, my friends," is a familiar salutation to those who, for more than thirty years, faithfully listened to my coast-to-coast radio and television nutrition programs. That greeting opened every one of more than thirty-one thousand such broadcasts that I did beginning in 1941.

It is both chastening and heartening to realize that I am now teaching nutrition to the grandchildren of my original listeners and readers—not only on the air and in books, but in lectures, seminars, and the classrooms of universities. It was only a few months ago that one of my college students remarked, "I hated you when I was a child. I was never allowed to have candy, chewing gum, cake, soda pop, or white bread. But I don't have a cavity in my mouth—so I guess you knew what you were talking about."

The incident recalled a serious suggestion from one of my early listeners and readers. She proposed that I create a lapel button to warn away grandparents and friends so oblivious to good nutrition as to visit with lollipops in hand.

The button was to read: "Fredericks child—don't feed!" (They give protection against the well-meaning but ignorant to the animals in the zoo, don't they?)

I remember a luncheon I once held for more than two hundred children and their parents, the children of families who had been infertile until my broadcasts and books persuaded them to rectify their diets. I shall always remember the beaming woman who, at that event, introduced me to her husband, explaining: "It's time, dear, that you met the father of our children." Which didn't exactly justify the remark host Mike Douglas made on the air: "Dr. Fredericks is the father of more than two hundred children!"—because he refused to explain!

The most frequent statement in the millions of letters I've received from listeners and readers is, "Why are the newspapers, magazines, TV, and new books making such a fuss about the 'recent discoveries' you told us about a quarter of a century ago?" To which my reply is a thought borrowed from Montaigne: When it's first discovered, it's not true. Twenty years later, it's true, but not important. After another thirty years it's true, it's important; but fifty years later, what are you getting upset about? That, of course, describes the inevitable cultural lags that separate the discovery, acceptance, and ultimate application of health findings that can help mankind. These unnecessary delays have caused unnecessary suffering.

In trying to shorten these cultural lags, I often in the past infuriated the nutrition establishment as I noted the enormous leverage the food industry—with its gross income of $125 billion a year—wields. Glenn Doman, celebrated for his research in patterning brain-injured children, remarked to me that I had done what he had done; I had violated the establishment's "territorial imperative."

Reprisals from the nutrition establishment avoided a discussion of the issues, and took shape, inevitably, as an attack on the man. It is easier to challenge the nutritionist's credentials and competence than to contrive a valid defense of poor foods, dubious additives, questionable pesticide residues, or white bread deprived of its fiber.

In refreshing contrast is the climate in nutrition today. Although I am not an M.D. but a Ph.D. (which, to the sugar-and-white-flour manufacturers, means "possibly half-demented"), I write now as the recently elected president of the International Academy of Preventive Medicine, as a member of the board of governors of another medical society, as a regular contributor to a medical journal, and as editor of a medical newsletter. My long-term listeners and readers remain wary, nonetheless! Hearing of this professional acceptance of my credentials and competence, a reader wrote, "They tried for thirty years to shut you up by excommunicating you, and it didn't work, so they're going to take you in, and *then* gag you."

Despite my reader's understandable reservations, the climate in nutrition *is* changing dramatically. I am now delivering papers and seminars in nutrition to thousands of physicians, dentists, biochemists, and nutritionists who, a few years ago, would have attended only if permitted to wear false beards. Thousands of physicians in the United States, in Canada, in South America, in Mexico, and abroad are now using nutrition as an adjunct (and frequently prime) therapy in their practices. Many psychiatrists have discarded the couch in favor of the dining table, and many analysts have discarded theories of toilet training and are practicing psychonutrition, with goodly doses of vitamins and other nutrients appended to corrected diet in the treatment of neurosis and psychosis.

The U.S. Department of Agriculture recently issued a monograph that states that 90 per cent of our sicknesses could be mitigated or wiped out merely by improvements in diet. These concessions are an acknowledgment that the grassroots movement in my field, so long contemptuously dismissed as "food faddism," has at last influenced the professional disciplines that for so many years neglected or mocked the claims made for improved nutrition. This proves the validity of the old New England aphorism that says we tend to be down on what we're not up on.

To you who are about to read this book on the high-fiber diet, an appeal: If this is your first contact with avant garde nutrition, don't let it be the last. Between the hyperbole of the cultist and the negativism of those who should be but aren't informed in nutrition, there is a middle ground. If you explore it, you may reap dividends that will astonish you.

The greatest reward, though, may be a negative one—what *doesn't* happen. This book is addressed to that middle ground, and to those negative dividends. The bowel cancer, appendicitis, diverticular disease, hemorrhoids, and varicose veins that you *don't* get are very real, very tangible rewards. I wish these rewards for you, and I am sorry that the cultural lag has deprived you of dietary protection against these diseases for such a long time.

—CARLTON FREDERICKS, PH.D., F.I.A.P.M.

Carlton Fredericks' High-Fiber Way to Total Health

1. We Must Be Doing Something Wrong

In the time it will take you to read this book, a dozen people in the United States will learn they have bowel cancer, and six patients with that disease will die. Those who survive longer may have colostomies—that is, operations to bypass the ravaged area of the bowel. Colostomies are so frequently performed that some victims have established a society to help newcomers learn how to live with the inconveniences, the embarrassment, and the emotional strains that accompany the life-saving surgery.

It never seems to occur to those patients, and undoubtedly it hasn't occurred to you, that bowel cancer and other serious disorders of the digestive tract can be *prevented*. They are not inescapable punishments dispensed by an irate Providence, but penalties for our biological insanity in selecting our foods.

This is *not* theory, for we have studied large groups of people from "primitive" cultures in parts of Africa who escape these diseases (and many others)—*until* they discard their time-tested diet for long-term use of "civilized" manufactured foods. Until then, these Africans simply don't develop our tooth decay, periodontal disease, constipation, diverticulosis, diverticulitis, polyps, hemorrhoids, appendicitis, varicose veins, and bowel cancer. And as for heart disease, the Africans' diet is a nightmare for cardiologists. Many Africans consume gargantuan amounts of high-cholesterol foods and yet remain so immune to coronary thrombosis that a case of it in rural Africa is considered to be a medical curiosity.

What precisely is protective about this African diet, and why does ours fail to shield us? Is the African who stays with his native diet avoiding something harmful that we consume, or do his foods provide something missing from ours? Where are the chinks in *our* nutritional armor?

Even a superficial study of African foods shows that many people in rural areas consume three times as much fiber as the average American. Those inexperienced in the complexities of human nutrition have seized upon this as *the* explanation for the African's immunities to many vascular and heart disorders as well as to digestive problems. *There is no doubt that our food is short of fiber, and that this deficiency is related to our susceptibility to a number of diseases*. But after forty years in the field of nutrition, I have learned to be wary of simplistic answers to questions involving the enormous complexities of the human body and its reactions to foods. I learned from Dr. Linus Pauling that the first critical step toward the training of a scientist begins when he learns to say, "I don't believe it."

I don't believe, for instance, that restoration of the proper kind and amount of fiber to our diet will wipe out coronary thrombosis. I make the prophecy that we will learn that the African's protection against heart disease is predicated upon factors *other* than his consumption of high-fiber foods, though the consumption of high-fiber foods may help. (See Chapters 14 and 15, which deal with heart disease.)

The lack of fiber in our own diet, however, certainly does slow down the passage of food residues from the body and does contribute to constipation, and thereby—as the evidence clearly shows—makes us easy targets for the digestive and blood-vessel diseases to which the Africans studied are so patently immune.

Fiber's History

Clues to dietary fiber were uncovered in the sixteenth century, when the properties of bran in helping elimination were first noticed. Then, many decades ago, Sir Robert McCarrison showed that animals fed a diet common to one region developed that region's prevalent diseases. The medical journals of McCarrison's day seized upon the astonishing discovery that poor nutrition could cause dysfunction and pathology of every system, tissue, and organ in the body—skin, nails, bones, eyes, brain, blood, heart, lymphatic system, muscles, stomach, intestines, liver, spleen, colon, and glands. But many ignored McCarrison's conclusion, which was even more important—that a good diet means good health.

Why do we hear more about disease than about good health? Maybe because doctors reflect our orientation toward sickness. Our doctors to this day sometimes seem vaguely uncomfortable when they tell us, "Go home—there is nothing wrong with you." It is as if they were uneasy in the presence of ·vell-being—perhaps because their experience with it is so limited.

Dr. Weston Price was one of the first men to study rural Africans before and after the introduction of westernized diet. Price's original interest was in tooth decay, but he soon found that our foods descended on Africa like a blight. Tooth decay was only the first in a long series of penalties for poor diet that even included birth defects. His comparisons of the nutritional values of the primitive diets anc the westernized menus that succeeded them were instructive. He showed that the unaltered native diet produced good health and shielded the African from the illnesses and deformities common among westerners. But Price's observations, like McCarrison's, remained hidden in nutritional archives, ignored by all but a handful of nutritionists and medical men interested in preventive medicine.

Our medical facilities are increasingly crowded with patients suffering from disorders of the heart, blood vessels, colon, and bowels. Western manufacturers of digitalis pills, laxatives, cathartics, mineral oil, psyllium powder, enemas, suppositories, antacids, and anti-spasmodics would go bankrupt in such unwesternized areas as Africa. The diet of the African is assuredly the protective factor, for his immunities disappear when he succumbs to the meretricious appeal of the foods of civilization—just as the Eskimo increases his susceptibility to diabetes after he is introduced to white sugar and raises his consumption of it beyond seventy pounds per year. (We eat a staggering one hundred twenty pounds of white sugar per person per year, and that contributes to many of the sicknesses discussed in this book.)

The Siren Call of Western Food

There have been many studies of the health ailments and diets of rural Africans, and for good reason.

Ischemic heart disease—exemplified by *coronary thrombosis*—is now responsible for a third of all deaths in the United States, but in Africa it was until recently virtually unknown. (Now it is beginning to increase, very slowly, in large cities.)

Appendicitis is the most frequent cause of abdominal emergency operations in our country. In Africa, it is virtually unknown in rural areas —but its incidence, like that of heart disease, is starting to rise in the communities that are becoming westernized.

Diverticular disease—ballooning of the segments of the walls of the colon—is, in the United States, regarded as the most common disease of that organ. In Africa, the medical experts term it "exceedingly rare."

Varicose veins, afflicting one in ten of us, occur in only one in a thousand rural Africans— but, again, the incidence of varicose veins is beginning to increase among those who adopt western customs.

Thrombosis (clots) of the deep veins and resulting *pulmonary embolism*, feared and frequent postoperative complications, are almost unknown in Africans who resist western customs.

Hiatus hernia, a very uncomfortable disorder, is a source of trouble for nearly half the American population over fifty years of age. It, too, is almost unknown in the rural African. So are

hemorrhoids, whereas the incidence of hemorrhoids in the United States is similar to that of
hiatus hernia.

Cancer of the colon and rectum is, in our
country, second only to lung cancer as a cause
of death from malignancies; it is rare in Africans.

The common note in all these reports, the re-
frain one encounters again and again, is: The
African escapes many of our disorders of the
digestive tract, the blood vessels, and the heart
if he remains deaf to the siren call of western
foods.

Was it instinct that guided these Africans to
select a diet that protected them against bowel
cancer and the other diseases in the long, mel-
ancholy list of digestive and vascular disorders
to which we in America are increasingly subject? It was not; and don't speculate about an
inner voice of "wisdom of the body" that dictated their food choices and rejections. "Inner
wisdom" would have warned them away from
our grocery stores!

The Africans' guide was inherited knowledge,
based upon centuries of experience, that was
handed down from one generation to the next.
That, obviously, couldn't equip them to appraise
our unnatural foods, which are irretrievably
altered by the western chemist, "seasoned" with
dubious additives and pesticide residues, and
deliberately overprocessed so that insects—

somehow aware that such foods will not support life—avoid them.

When rural people such as Africans fall prey to the "convenience" of westernized foods, it's only a matter of time before many become victims of such disorders as sluggishness of the bowel, constipation, and, ultimately, digestive diseases, vascular diseases—and bowel cancer. Let's consider why.

2. If It Will Keep, Throw It Out— If It Will Spoil, Eat It Before It Does

As the deep-sea fish will be the last to "discover" salt water, so is it unlikely that you're aware of the sheer strangeness of the foods you consume. Take the experiment in which monkeys were fed on a selection of foods that came high on the average American shopping list and were popularly regarded as the basis of a balanced diet. The objective was a study of the processes leading to atherosclerosis (hardening of the arteries). The monkeys died before atherosclerosis could develop! It has not yet been announced what the researchers found—in a typical American diet, remember—that killed them.

Consider the fact that perhaps half the foods you eat were not in existence thirty years ago (and, I hope, will not be two decades from now). Reflect on the fact that pigs are optimally fed by giving them nutrient-packed residues—that is, what's left after the non-nutritive ingredients of white flour (which *you* eat) have been removed.* And don't believe it's only our wheat that is raped rather than reaped. Consider the implications of this statement by a researcher who has been investigating the body's reaction to rice bran (like wheat bran, a residue of over-processing): "Rice bran has been shown to dramatically lower serum-, liver-, and aorta-cholesterol levels by 33 per cent to 50 per cent." Helping the body to excrete cholesterol in this way may be saner than manipulating the diet in an effort to avoid intake of cholesterol, which is, after all, necessary for life and health.

Why do the processors do what they do? Because they are not as interested in retention of nutritional values as they are in a product's long shelf life. The two are usually mutually exclusive, because only bad food "keeps." We have an old axiom in nutrition: If it will keep, throw it out; if it will spoil, eat it before it does. This doctrine automatically bans from the diet white flour, polished rice, and other devitalized grains that contribute greatly to digestive and vascular disorders because of their deficiencies in fiber and in important nutrients.

The processor wants a saleable, palatable product, one that is easy to prepare, easy to chew (or doesn't require chewing at all), and one, preferably, that need not be dated for freshness.

---

* Industry critics of this statement should read the *Mill Feeds Manual*, obtainable from the Wheat Flour Institute, an organization, oddly, devoted to shielding white flour from (richly deserved) criticism.

And remember that part of the responsibility for all this is on your shoulders. You don't buy foods on the basis of the needs of your body, but on the basis of habit, price, convenience, the conditioning of advertising, and the pleasures of the (slightly jaded) palate. And when you stop to think about it, you very well know that your selections are poor. Why else would you hesitate to feed your table scraps to a valuable pedigreed dog, or to permit your infant to participate in the adult meals?

Are We Healthy Now?

While I'm making an effort to anticipate blocks in your acceptance of the thesis of this book, which links our diet to our common sicknesses, let me disabuse you of the illusion that "We must be well-fed—after all, we're living longer, and we're a lot healthier than other nations." Here are a few statistics given by Dr. W. D. Currier, of the International Academy of Metabology, Inc., in his presidential message to the physician-membership.

"The United States has dropped from seventh in the world to sixteenth in the prevention of infant mortality. It has dropped in female life expectancy from sixth to eighth. It has dropped in male life expectancy from tenth to twenty-fourth. And it has bought itself this unenviable trend by spending more of its gross national product for medical care (a dollar of every fourteen dollars) than any other country on the face of the earth."

Isn't it obvious that the answers are not to be found in pills, powders, capsules, injections, elixirs, syrups, ointments, surgery, chemotherapy, and radiation treatment? Isn't it time to look at this patent fact: *When we export our food, we export many of our sicknesses*? Isn't it time for us to escape being targets for crisis medicine, and to become examples of prevention?

BAMBY

Our efforts to acquire the immunities of the Africans should take advantage of everything their experience can teach us. If you carefully study the scientific literature deriving from studies of primitive diet—and carefully read *Nutrition and Physical Degeneration* by Weston Price—you will arrive at a program that I call, with no apologies to Walt Disney, the BAMBY plan. BAMBY is an acronym to help you remember these nutritional protections:

> Bran
> And
> Multiple vitamins and minerals
> B-complex vitamins
> Yogurt

The BAMBY plan can be shaped into criteria for food selection, recipe composition, and menu makeup.

Inertia is inappropriate in a reader of a book such as this. But, knowing human nature, I have arranged the BAMBY plan so that you may either adopt it wholeheartedly and totally revise your dietary habits, or take the path of least resistance and use bran tablets, B-complex capsules or liquids, and concentrates of "friendly" bacteria in tablet form.*

Whatever your state of health—whether you're well and want to stay that way, or overweight and want to lose, or already have one of the "civilized" diseases and wish (under medical direction) to arrest it before it progresses any further—the BAMBY plan makes *health sense.*

---

* Since bran may increase excretion of certain minerals, a multiple mineral supplement is protective.

3. Constipation—Is It "Normal"?

The journey from digestive health to digestive disease often begins with constipation. It may seem to be a minor disorder, but it may signal a life-threatening disease, for it is associated with profound changes in the function and the chemistry of the colon and bowel.

Somehow, physicians have tended to be more impressed by diarrhea than by constipation. A persistent case of diarrhea may seem like more of a challenge to the medical man, even when it is likely that the sufferer is a traveler returning from Mexico and the victim of nothing more than a mild case of Montezuma's Revenge. A persistent case of constipation, though, may elicit nothing more from your doctor than a short lecture on the importance of establishing a regular time for elimination, of avoiding straining, and, perhaps, of taking a stool-softener or lubricating oil, laxative, suppository, cathartic, or enema. It is not good medical practice, however, merely to relieve the symptoms of constipation, for its origin is uncertain—and its occurrence could indicate something is direly wrong.

Some practitioners may decide that constipation is normal, on the grounds that they encounter many healthy people who have bowel movements only once every three or four days, or even only once a week. These doctors have arrived at the misleading conclusion that "average" is healthy. It isn't. If you have fallen into the trap of that kind of logic, consider that loosening and loss of teeth occur in 80 per cent of Americans after the age of thirty-five. It's average—but certainly not healthy.

Nevertheless, medical men will scold patients for being too preoccupied with frequency of evacuation. "You will become needlessly laxative-dependent," they warn. "There is no need for a daily movement. Many healthy people don't have them." (And how many of these healthy people become medical statistics later?)

Constipation alone isn't the entire problem in digestive disorders, though it plays an important part. Faulty diets cause another undesirable phenomenon—prolonged stool-transit time. This is merely the medical way of saying that the exodus of food wastes from the body is abnormally delayed. Constipation and prolonged stool-transit time are not necessarily concomitant, but frequently are.

A third aspect of the problem is stool bulk. When proper steps are taken to cope with constipation and to adjust the stool-transit time to normal, the bulk of the stool tends to be reduced when it is too great and to be enlarged when it is too small. When the diet is healthful the changes will be healthful. But healthful adjustments in stool bulk are rare phenomena in a country which has not yet learned that fast foods may be slow death!

4.   Food Residues and Bacteria

To understand digestive disorders—their problems and their solutions—it is helpful to take a worm's-eye view of what happens to food after you've chewed and swallowed it. Its initial destination is the stomach. There, your food is churned with acid and with digestive enzymes that begin the process of breaking it down into its constituents. The body (with good reason not trusting your choices) will later assemble these into the compounds that meet its nutritional needs.

Contrary to the popular concept, absorption of food and its constituents isn't a prime function of the stomach. Absorption takes place all the way from the mouth to the rectal exit. If that astonishes you, remember that there are medications given sublingually (under the tongue) that are promptly absorbed, and that the drugs in rectal suppositories readily enter the body from the lower bowel.

Exiting from the stomach (and on occasion probably leaving it in a state of disbelief), your churned and predigested food enters the small intestine, so called because of its small diameter, not its length, which is over twenty feet. Here food is treated with other digestive substances needed to break it down; these originate principally in the liver and the pancreas.

The small intestine is a miracle of anatomical engineering, for the absorption surfaces there would, if rolled out flat, cover more than half a basketball court. The majority of the nutritional elements in your foods reach the body through the walls of the small intestine. Then, by the rippling conga dance the medical man calls "peristalsis," the residue is extruded, like ointment from a large tube, into the colon—the large intestine. Here the body manages somehow to separate liquid and solid. The intestinal wall absorbs excess fluid after the solid portion of the stool has journeyed toward the rectum.

Bacterial Flora

A very important phenomenon has occurred during this journey of the food residues. Bacteria normal to ⁺he large bowel have been added to the stool—indeed, they now constitute a large part of the weight and bulk of it. These bacteria come from your "bacterial flora"—a term I have used with diffidence ever since one of my university students said he would like to meet her!

Both the food residues and the intestinal bacteria have long invited from the public what physicians have considered to be a neurotic preoccupation. People for generations have used innumerable medications to "clean out the bowel," and to stamp out the bacteria. Since the enormous bacterial concentration in the large intestine was viewed as a kind of smoldering infection, it was blamed for "auto-intoxication," a condition of self-poisoning causing a complex of vague symptoms. To cope with this, the public enthusiastically resorted to high colonics, oral (and anal!) doses of yogurt, and tablets of compressed "friendly bacteria." The medical profession took a dim view of the theory and the treatment, but the followers of this school of thought were closer to the truth than the medical cynics believed.

If the food we eat is so highly overprocessed that it doesn't yield enough natural residue to stimulate elimination, not only will constipation result, but the transit time for the stool in its progress through the bowel will be prolonged. That lingering process gives added opportunity for the gut bacteria to attack certain chemicals normally produced by the body as part of the digestive process and normally excreted with the stool. The compounds that result when those chemicals are broken down are known to be powerful and effective triggers of cancer.

This, then, is the mechanism by which we postulate that prolonged stool-transit time and constipation become vectors of cancer of the bowel. The disease is not produced by a mistake of nature, for what happens is the product of unnatural reactions to unnatural foods. Nature doesn't make starches and sugars devoid of fiber, nor does she strip them of vitamins, minerals, and fats. We must take the responsibility for the mischief perpetrated by white flour, white sugar, white rice, degerminated corn, overmilled rye, and overprocessed barley. Not only are these foods that "keep" (a property we've already labelled as suspect), but when we eat them, we tend to keep the unnatural residues within us long enough for trouble to begin.

The studies of primitive Africans show that these people stay healthy because their diets stimulate elimination, which is to say that their starches and sugars are unmilled, unfractionated, high in bran and fiber, rich in vitamins and minerals. The primitive African obeys the laws of nature, and remains healthy unless we change his internal environment with our westernized foods.

5. Digestive Disorders

When the testing of atom bombs was contaminating the atmosphere with radioactive strontium 90, native peoples in the far north were particularly jeopardized. They feed on the caribou, which feed on moss. The moss acted as a sponge, absorbing and concentrating the strontium 90 that fell with the rain, with the result that the Eskimos and Indians of the region, consuming caribou meat liberally seasoned with the deadly strontium 90, were carrying a heavy body burden of radioactivity.

The suggestion was made that we place the Eskimos and Indians on our diet of processed foods. Because of the excessive processing to which much of our food is subjected, the strontium-90 content of these peoples' diets would be lowered significantly—and so would the nutritional values of those diets. The suggestion was rejected, *Time* magazine noted, because "our diet would fall upon primitives as a blight."

When we inflict that blight on primitives, we not only deprive them of fiber and the potent biological values of the grain germ—we also deprive them of essential vitamins and minerals.

We manage to alter the bacterial life in their guts until it resembles ours. The implications of this were not apparent until recently, for we know very little about the microbial life within the human bowel—in fact, it has seriously been said that any scientist wh thinks he can fully understand the functions of bowel bacteria in even one type of mammal should be tucked away in a mental institution. (That cynical remark isn't based just on what we don't know about the teeming life in the human bowel. It also reflects the contradictions in what little we *do* know about it, for there is much evidence that refuses to fit logically into any overall theory that makes sense.)

We've always regarded the bowel as more or less the "holding tank" for digestive residues. This idea meant that both the nature and the activities of bowel microbes sho ld not be nutritionally significant, even though the number of bacteria was so great that about 30 per cent of the weight of the stool consisted of these organisms. Yet any physician who has prescribed long-term oral doses of antibiotics that are aimed at infections but are known to attack our "normal" bowel bacteria, too, has seen an occasional patient who develops a sore tongue or other symptoms of deficiency in the B vitamins. There are even reports that some of these patients develop classic deficiency diseases—pellagra, for instance. It is for this reason that some manufacturers began to advise doctors to help restore "friendly" bowel bacteria by prescribing frequent doses of yogurt or concentrated tablets of lactobacilli when oral antibiotics were to be taken for more than five or six days.

In depleting our gut bacteria, is the antibiotic depriving us of essential vitamins that we know they synthesize? Perhaps, but we're not supposed to depend on that small and uncertain source for our vitamins; the absorption from the bowel, in any case, shouldn't be that critical for us. Even if gut bacteria in some way facilitate the absorption of vitamins from food, why would bacteria-killing antibiotics have a significant effect when the bulk of vitamins is absorbed from the small intestine, many feet away from the bowel, and (normally) bacteria-free? Answers are certainly not yet available, but we logically conclude that the *living organisms in the lower end of the gut are important in ways not yet understood,* and interfering with them can be a definite threat to health.

Bowel Cancer

When stool-transit time is slow and/or constipation is present—and both of these disorders are intimately associated with the American low-fiber diet that is so sparsely supplied with the vitamin B complex—the bowel bacteria may get their opportunity to attack and to change chemically the composition of the stool.

To understand what happens, you should realize that the stool contains, in each day's accumulation of food residues, perhaps a pint of bile.* Bile is a greenish fluid that is essential for the digestion of fats, for the utilization of fat-soluble vitamins, and for an initial step in the digestion of protein. Bile is produced in diluted form in the liver, and becomes more highly concentrated in the gall bladder.

Normal bile contains two acids. Their names aren't important, but their chemical structures are, *for both acids can be changed into cancer-producing (carcinogenic) compounds by the action of intestinal bacteria.* This effect becomes possible when stool-transit time is unnaturally slow, as it is in people who eat low-fiber diets. Because the stool traverses the intestine lethargically and lingers in the bowel, the bacteria are given time to convert the bile acids from harmless chemicals essential to digestion into carcinogens. The same delay permits these potent cancer inciters to remain in prolonged and intimate contact with the vulnerable soft tissues of the gut. In this bath of carcinogens, the tissue will gradually undergo changes, proceeding from premalignancy to outright cancer. Rural Africans on high-fiber diets almost never get

---

* Some of this is reabsorbed by the body; some is excreted with the food residues.

bowel cancer because stool-transit time is accelerated and constipation is rare.

These factors, though, aren't the only sources of the Africans' immunities to bowel cancer. There is also evidence that the *nature* of their gut bacteria is different—primarily because their foods are different from ours. This is not based on speculation, for we know that *high-fiber diets* fed to Americans will change the bacterial flora and raise the excretion of *unaltered* bile acids. Conversely, on *low-fiber diets*, Americans excrete less-than-usual amounts of these acids in their original chemical form, indicating that *the acids have changed into other compounds.**

We can see the process at work in black Americans. Genetically, they are kin to the Africans we have studied, but they do not share their immunities. American blacks house bowel bacteria of the type that *can* break down bile acids, and, as a result, the American descendant of the African native has the same incidence of bowel cancer as our white population. Americans, regardless of color or ancestry, have nine to thirteen times as much cancer of the bowel as occurs in the African natives on their time-honored, century-tested diets.

----

* One alternative theory indicts a high-fat, high-beef diet for enzyme changes conducive to bowel cancer. This doesn't negate the value of raising fiber intake from the low level of the American diet.

The Influence of Heredity

To say that studies of the relationship between gut bacteria and health are easier in animals than in man is probably to make the understatement of the scientific century. It is possible to breed animals that are completely free of bacteria, and we know that such animals will excrete unchanged chemicals that, exposed to the usual bacterial flora, would be converted into carcinogens. Such studies in humans would not be easy to make!

Independent of what happens with dietary fiber, bacterial flora, stool-transit time, and constipation is the influence of heredity on our enzyme chemistries. A topical example of a genetically controlled response to dietary factors is found in reactions to the artificial sweetener cyclamate. You have undoubtedly read diametrically opposed reports in which this sugar-substitute is described (on the one hand) as perfectly safe or (on the other) as a carcinogenic factor. Part of the confusion derives from the fact that some people—not all—have an enzyme system that breaks down the cyclamate molecule, releasing a component that is weakly carcinogenic. This is not directly relevant to the thesis of this book, but it emphasizes the importance of approaching our health problems realistically.

We can't do much about genetically dictated enzyme systems that may trigger adverse reactions outside of avoiding substances that might initiate such consequences. But we can and *must* do something about changing our dietary habits to rid ourselves of purely gratuitous and life-threatening hazards—particularly when we know what incredible health dividends may accrue from a few simple changes in our food habits.

Prevention

In talking with hundreds of medical nutritionists at seminars and conventions, and in reading the spate of recent books and scientific papers on the subject of fiber in the diet, I find the emphasis is almost exclusively on the prevention of bowel cancer, appendicitis, diverticular disease, and the other serious sicknesses that may be avoided with sufficient intake of fiber. While the emphasis on prevention is refreshing, it is analogous to discussing vitamin-C deficiency only in terms of scurvy.

Deficiency of a vitamin may not be life-threatening, but it does attack well-being. For instance, total lack of vitamin B_1 can cause beriberi—a disease that kills. But partial deficiency will cause trouble too—lethargy, nervousness, irritability, and unjustified feelings of anxiety. By the same token, "ordinary constipation" certainly doesn't threaten you with immediate, serious disease. But it can nonetheless cause a constellation of symptoms that will take the fun out of living, interfere with both physical and mental functioning, and keep you running from psychiatrist to allergist to gastroenterologist or internist.

For years, observing physicians have commented on constipated patients who feel distinctly better, physically and mentally, when they use laxatives, cathartics, or high colonics. Merely raising their intake of fruits and vegetables, the doctors often note, doesn't elicit a response in such patients. It is useful in this regard to note that recent evidence indicates that cereal fiber is much more effective in relieving constipation than fiber from vegetables and fruits.

A gastroenterologist who has written a classic textbook on digestive disorders remarks that many patients with "ordinary constipation" have many other, related symptoms that, unfortunately, are not usually charged to the lethargy of the intestinal tract or the toxic effect of constipation on the liver. Some of these people suffer from depression that is clearly endogenous— i.e., unrelated to their life situations, and of internal origin. Others complain of disturbances of the eye muscles, of headaches and dizziness, of infections of teeth, tonsils, and sinuses, of allergies, of chronic, low-grade inflammation of the intestinal tract. The specialist diagnoses such patients as reacting systemically to the type of bacteria inhabiting their bowels, *despite the fact* that these organisms are usually described as harmless. We must remember, of course, that "harmfulness" is often caused by the body's lack of resistance, and is not necessarily a characteristic of an organism; but the point is that the effects of a digestive disturbance can be much more far-reaching than the average person—or doctor—supposes.

The gastroenterologist also comments on the fact that a "harmless" streptococcus germ of the type common in the bowels of Americans will, when injected into animals, cause gall-bladder disturbances, joint pains, and, in a small percentage, heart, blood-vessel, and nervous-system lesions. Thus we can see that "harmless" bacteria are not always harmless, and that they must be kept in control—that is, functioning in the way nature intended them to.

6. Yogurt

What I said before will have a familiar ring to those of us who know of Ilya Ilyich Metchnikoff; he was the man who attributed the superb health and long life spans of Bulgarians to their high intake of yogurt and other fermented milk products that are rich sources of "friendly" bacteria. He felt that the yogurt-eaters were avoiding self-poisoning by constantly implanting "friendly" bacteria in their bowels. "Self-poisoning" was translated into "auto-intoxication"; this became a catch-phrase that persuaded millions of people to consume kefir, koumiss, and yogurt in an effort to change the bacterial flora of the gut.

There is no particular significance in the fact that orthodox medicine rejected the concept of auto-intoxication, for it also initially rejected vitamins, the electroencephalogram, penicillin, fever thermometers and smallpox vaccination. Nevertheless, the theory of auto-intoxication is still listed in some medical textbooks as an example of the fads to which the public and some physicians have fallen prey in the past. Now, a half century later, we find the concept, supported by new evidence, returning, as high-fiber diets and sources of beneficial micro-organisms, like yogurt, become part of a dietary defense against some of civilization's common diseases.

Medical orthodoxy, be it clearly understood, still does not embrace the auto-intoxication concept with enthusiasm. It has in the past made a number of attempts to downgrade the value of yogurt, exactly as it has denied the value of and the need for vitamin-and-mineral supplements. The American Medical Association (A.M.A.) has said yogurt offers nothing more than the benefits of ordinary milk—at a much higher price. However, René Dubos, of the Rockefeller Institute, demonstrated that implanting yogurt-type "friendly" bacteria in the bowels of animals resulted in heightened resistance to infection as well as a lengthened life span.

Reporting on his findings, Dubos remarked, "Walking in Metchnikoff's footsteps once more, we are inclined to believe that the usual intestinal flora are an expression of man's total environment, and that their control may turn out to have as profound effects on the well-being of human infants and adults as it has on the growth of mice and of farm animals."

After René Dubos' paper appeared in 1962, the *Journal* of the A.M.A. published a quasi-apologetic editorial (unfortunately largely unseen by the public, which *had* read the widely publicized criticisms of "yogurt faddism"). The editorial admitted the possibility that Dubos' findings showed a need for a reassessment of the values of yogurt-type organisms in supporting better health. The Rockefeller research thereby supplies part of the background for the recommendation that the high-fiber, low-sugar diet be made more effective by the use of a source of yogurt-type "friendly" bacteria.

7. If It's Good for You, It's Not Popular

Removal of fiber from our overprocessed foods means simultaneous depletion of a number of B-complex vitamins and trace minerals—vitamins and minerals that are as important to normal liver function as they are to the health of the colon and bowel. In the grain germ, which is the wheat seed's embryo and the source from which the new life sprouts, nature has concentrated vital vitamin B-complex and mineral values.* These are as important as fiber in helping you to achieve disease immunities.

If yours is an average American market basket, half its calories will come from sugar, wheat, rice, buckwheat, corn, and barley products—as manufactured cereals, flour, snack foods, and baked products. The latter are *all* monuments to departed fiber and discarded vitamin-and-mineral values. The residues, it has been noted, may be converted into pig feed—or

---

* Wheat germ, like most grain embryos, contains a fair amount of fiber, too.

mink feed. Minks, which have a high cash value, are *very* carefully fed.

This peculiar "civilized" system of value judgments about food is applied to meat purchases, too. The organ meats, like liver and kidneys, which are richer in nutrients and less costly than the muscle meats (steaks, chops, and roasts) are largely ignored. One can almost say: If it's good for you, it's not popular. There certainly is an American ritual built about liver; it's eaten once a week, if at all. Eating it twice might trigger a visit by a government agency dedicated to stamping out food faddism!

Our habits with fruits and vegetables violate the laws of biology, too. We drink fruit juices, and they are usually strained, apparently so we can avoid the fiber of the pulp. (We can avoid the exercise of *chewing* with strained juices, and this allows us to buy water-massage machines twenty years later in an effort to save deteriorating gums and loosening teeth.) We carefully peel vegetables and fruits, again minimizing fiber intake. Doesn't the skin of the baked potato more often reach the garbage bag than the gastrointestinal tract?

What a *Low-Fiber* Diet Does to You

We have identified the ways in which our low-fiber diet alters colon function, contributing to slow stool-transit time and constipation. (It should be emphasized that the absence of constipation does not mean that the transit time is necessarily ideal. Even with daily bowel movements, your Monday evacuation may be the one you should have had on Saturday.) We have also traced to the American low-fiber diet actions of the bacterial flora in the bowel that can launch a series of toxic effects associated with constipation. We have seen, in fact, that a low-fiber diet can cause the beginning of degenerative changes in the soft tissues of the bowel—changes that can—and often do—lead to bowel cancer.

But these are only some of the realizations that shock you as you study "primitive" immunity versus "civilized" sickness. The packed colon and bowel associated with fiber deficiency can contribute to varicose veins, deep thrombosis of the veins, hemorrhoids (which are actually varicose veins), and diverticular disease. And when large amounts of sugar are taken in the low-fiber diet—and this is the usual western pattern of eating—the toll of the low-fiber diet will include tooth decay and periodontal diseases. Periodontal diseases—disorders of the supporting structures of the teeth—may originate in part with sugar's effect on glandular function and in part with the lack of exercise for teeth, gums, and jawbone that comes with the softness and mushiness of the foods that are characteristic of a low-fiber diet.

8. Sugar, Sugar, and More Sugar!

It isn't just lack of fiber in grain-based foods that does all the mischief. It is also the ease with which such foods—and sugar—are over-consumed. If you eat five ounces of sugar a day—and for some people that quantity (equal to about forty teaspoonfuls) is low—you are consuming the equivalent of over two pounds of the sugar beet from which the sweetener was extracted and concentrated. And in the normal order of nutritional matters, as the authorities point out, no one would dream of eating two pounds of sugar beet!

An example given by Dr. Thomas L. Cleave, making the same point, compares the consumption of twenty apples at one sitting to eating a quantity of candy providing about the same amount of sugar. Eating the candy or taking the equivalent amount of sugar in soda pop is part of the nutritional practice of millions of Americans. But how about the twenty apples? Would not even Adam lose his capacity after three or four? Obviously the form in which sugar reaches us, as Americans, is abnormal—not only in the sense that essential nutrients are removed by overprocessing, but in the sense that overconcentration of sugar permits—indeed, encourages—overconsumption. And that really lifts the lid of Pandora's Box and releases a swarm of plagues.

Overweight is an invention of man, a product of highly processed foods containing a high concentration of carbohydrates. You don't see obesity in animals in the wild, but it *is* inflicted on our pets when we are unkind enough to expose them to our faulty concepts of what constitutes good nutrition.

Obesity is associated with both hypertension and diabetes. Diabetes increases susceptibility to cancer of many types, and to heart attacks—witness that the Eskimos' troubles started when their intake of sugar reached about seventy pounds per person per year. Consequences do not appear overnight; it takes about twenty years for the incidence of diabetes in primitive groups previously virtually immune to it to begin to climb toward our level.

Low Blood Sugar

When we combine lack of fiber and vitamin B complex with high intake of sugar, we may initially drive the pancreas into excessive activity, flooding the body with too much insulin. Injections of insulin are deliberately administered to cause shock in the mentally ill, and those who overproduce insulin create in themselves a constant condition of near-shock. The trouble starts when the unnatural concentration of sugar in the blood—a result of the unnatural amount of it in our diets—drives bloodsugar (glucose) levels up too rapidly, forcing the body into excessive measures to keep bloodsugar levels down where they belong. When the body's reaction is excessive, low blood sugar results—caused, paradoxically, by *too much* sugar in the diet.

The condition is aggravated by caffeine and intensified by stress. Its symptoms include unprovoked anxiety, claustrophobia, a peculiar type of insomnia, frigidity in women and impotence in men, suicidal depression unrelated to actual life situations, maniacal outbursts of temper abnormal to the personality, and a craving for sweets, which is sometimes perverted into a craving for alcohol or drugs.*

The remedy for low blood sugar is a low-sugar diet—a diet that should also omit beverages containing caffeine, including tea, coffee, cocoa, and chocolate and cola drinks. Emphasis in such a diet should be placed on the intake of proteins, fats, and high-fiber carbohydrates that supply starch rather than sugar.

When neglected, as it often is because its

---

* There are physicians who deny that low blood sugar causes mental symptoms. Such medical myopia characterizes those who have not learned to recognize this condition.

symptoms are so suggestive of neurosis, hypoglycemia (low blood sugar) is a prelude to diabetes and, therefore, to the chain of ills that can result from *that* disease. In diabetes, the oversensitized, overresponsive pancreas ultimately becomes exhausted and shifts from manufacture of excessive amounts of insulin to inadequate production. This is an oversimplified explanation of diabetes—some people manage to exhibit both disorders simultaneously (diabetes with high blood sugar, with intermittent periods of low blood sugar)—but the basic sequence is from low blood sugar with too-high production of insulin to high blood sugar with too-low production or impaired utilization of insulin.

9. Our Unnatural Foods Are Making Us Ill

Very significant is the association of diverticulosis and diverticulitis with some other disorders that can be traced to diet. The low-fiber, high-sugar diet is a prelude not only to diverticulosis, but to appendicitis, gall-bladder inflammation or gallstones or both, diabetes, abdominal hernia, varicose veins, duodenal ulcer. When diseases cluster in this fashion, the scientist is driven to look for common—or at least overlapping—causes.

Mention of duodenal ulcer will arouse objections in the medical community and among a public so long conditioned to the concept that stomach and duodenal ulcers are "wound-stripes" of civilization and thereby mirror the stresses to which we are subjected. We are indebted to Dr. Thomas L. Cleave for a fascinating anecdote from the records of German army doctors at the Russian front in World War II. Psychiatrists then—and now—would certainly predict that gastric ulcers would appear more frequently in soldiers in the front lines who live constantly under the stress of imminent injury or death. The corollary would follow: Such ulcers would appear infrequently in the rear echelons, and still less frequently in the supply and administrative divisions that are hundreds of miles from the threat of dismemberment and death.

The opposite was revealed by the German studies. The incidence of gastric ulcers *rose* as the soldiers moved *away* from the front. For this, Cleave offers a logical explanation. The ill-supplied front-line troops were living "off the land," commandeering the food supplies of the Russian peasants, and thus were on a diet of crude, unrefined foods. The rear-echelon troops had increasing access to the "civilized" foods that were available at a reasonable distance from the front lines. The greater the distance the soldiers were from the front, the closer they were to Germany and its noodles, pastries, sweets, and western diet. The German soldier in battle, on the other hand, was eating "frozen vegetables, sour bread, and raw turnip." He was deprived of his accustomed food and, thereby, of his ulcer attacks.

The Truth

Science is an arena in which differences of opinion clash. From the tatters of theory demolished in whole or in part is the fabric of truth ultimately woven. One might expect, therefore, that observations about primitive Africans' immunity, westerners' susceptibilities, and dietary differences between the two cultures could be explained and justified in different—and frequently mutually exclusive—ways. Actually, all the theories agree; all indict the "civilized" diet with its accompanying spectacular incidence of gastric, colonic, and circulatory diseases, and all unite in crediting "primitive" foods with the protection enjoyed by the African groups.

From there on, however, the authorities differ. One medical authority blames varicose veins on straining at stool, which places severe pressure on the colon (resulting, incidentally, in diverticular disease) and on critical blood vessels, thereby causing the varicose veins and hemorrhoids. Another finds these disorders to be caused by the slight but constant and abnormal pressure of the colon on the venous system that comes with the slow passage of the stool associated with a low-fiber diet. A third authority points to our bowel bacterial flora as a culprit in disorders like gall-bladder syndrome, which he regards as the results of low-grade infections and inflammations that, in turn, are toxic reactions to bowel bacteria.

The common abdominal emergency, appendicitis, is likewise attributed to different causes, but all are based ultimately on the low-fiber diet replete with sugar. In one explanation, the dry stool, which has lost much of its water in its prolonged journey through the colon, drops a fecalith—literally, a little pebble—into the opening to the appendix and blocks it. Another theory postulates that the lethargic colon allows bacteria to multiply and the result is an infection of the appendix.

I have some reservations about both these explanations of appendicitis. For one thing, I remember a discussion of the reason for a higher incidence of appendicitis in males than in females; it revolved about a difference in the circulation of the blood in the appendix, that in the male's appendix being less efficient. But there is absolutely no doubt that appendicitis is rarer as fiber content in the diet is higher.

It matters not to us whose version of the anatomy of the problem is right. What is important can be stated simply: Our unnatural foods are making us ill. The logic of the situation demands that we begin to select our diet with the same sanity primitives do, remembering that they share our illnesses only when they share our foods.

10. Bran—Nutritional Superstar

Among avant garde nutritionists there has long been a philosophy that white bread is excellent for cleaning lampshades and suede shoes, that sugar is useful as a pesticide for garden nematodes, and that corn flakes and puffed rice make good packing materials for shipping fragile articles. Their only debit is that they aren't fit to eat.

It is somewhat comforting to find these realistic viewpoints, not very long ago dismissed contemptuously as food faddism, now adopted by enthusiastic proponents of the high-fiber diet. It is, however, disconcerting to read recent advertisements in which a giant cereal manufacturer extolls the importance of bran to health—disconcerting considering that this one company sells about $325 million worth of cereal yearly, and about $324 million worth of this is products that have had their bran, germ, vitamins, and minerals removed!

It is also distressing to realize that many physicians and dieticians, unable to shake off decades of indoctrination by the milling, baking, sugar, and cereal industries, still recommend white bread, corn flakes, and polished rice as acceptable—even good—foods.

I pause to note that an anonymous nutritionist for the A.M.A. recently listed my cookbook as "not recommended" on the specific grounds that the recipes emphasize "faddist" ingredients —such as whole grains, wheat germ, and, of course, bran. On the other hand, I'm delighted to find that a psychiatrist has praised the health virtues of high-fiber diets, for most analysts attribute colon disorders to a gut reaction to your spouse or mother-in-law, and a stomach ulcer to "what's eating you."

Unfortunately, the recent converts do not actually understand the nature of bran, however much they praise it. I have scanned current books in which physicians describe bran as "inert fiber," which, they assure us, is not only harmless but has previously unsuspected beneficial actions in warding off numerous diseases. It *is* beneficial, but it certainly *isn't* inert. It is a storehouse of nutritional values that are subtracted from white-flour products; it *isn't* roughage; and its values and benefits are certainly not *newly* appreciated. In my first book, published in 1941, I placed emphasis on the health benefits of whole grains that have the fiber and germ intact—and the advice wasn't new even *then*.

Vitamin B$_6$

For cogent reasons, bran deserves closer inspection. Far from being a mechanical broom for the bowel and nothing more, bran is surprisingly high in *protein*. It contains a *natural antibiotic* that may explain the heightened resistance to intestinal infection demonstrated by animals maintained on whole wheat.

Bran is also a rich source of vitamin B$_6$, a vitamin that bread should supply generously— and doesn't, thanks to the processing that removes the bran and germ. Deficiency in vitamin B$_6$, even when intermittent, has caused premalignant changes in the liver tissue of experimental animals. Coupled with *magnesium,* also supplied by bran, vitamin B$_6$ has been used effectively to reduce the tendency in human beings to kidney stones of the calcium oxalate type.

Vitamin B$_6$ deficiency has been found to be responsible for massive water storage in the tissues. It is a wonder more Americans don't have this condition, for vitamin B$_6$, which also affects heart function, is very sparsely supplied by our diet. Our bran-less and germ-less white bread has lost about 70 per cent of its original content of the vitamin!

Bran also contains *choline, pantothenic acid,*

and *manganese*. These are vital to the body's synthesis of *acetylcholine*. Acetylcholine is indispensable to the muscles, including those that make the colon and bowel function, and it also has many other functions.

Pantothenic acid has been used to treat regional ileitis, another of our very serious diseases of the colon, for which surgery—drastic and sometimes dangerous—has been the usual recourse. The importance of pantothenic acid in intestinal function is underlined by its postoperative use to help patients minimize retention of gas and to relieve intestinal lethargy and abdominal distention—all common aftereffects of abdominal surgery. Dr. Roger Williams, the pioneer biochemist-nutritionist who isolated and synthesized pantothenic acid, has repeatedly urged more study of the usefulness of this vitamin in the treatment and prevention of constipation.

All this emphasizes the importance to the digestive tract of a source of pantothenic acid, such as bran or wheat germ—and it underlines the hidden impact of food processing on our health. It has been discovered by the Japanese that the methyl bromide used to fumigate bran changes the pantothenic acid in it to another, *inactive* compound. This is just a single example of the insidious way in which our food is tampered with!

Bran Is Not Roughage

To consider bran as roughage is to perpetuate the misconception that banned it from the diet in intestinal disorders, like diverticular disease, that are actually caused by *lack* of fiber in the diet. *Bran is capable of absorbing many times its weight in water,* and in the body it therefore becomes bulkage, a lubricating type of "softage"; but it is not roughage. The bulkage provided by bran makes for the larger but softer stool now regarded as one of the sources of the Africans' immunities to many of our digestive disorders.

Bran is a source of *copper, iodine, iron, phosphorus, zinc,* and *trace amounts of other minerals important in human nutrition.* Don't dismiss these arbitrarily because of the small amounts involved. They add up—particularly when they're routinely *removed* from the carbohydrates that supply half the calories in the average diet. That lesson was learned dramatically by at least one hundred schizophrenics who are now functioning normally, thanks to a medical biochemist who gave them doses of zinc, vitamin B_6, and manganese. It is interesting to note that schizophrenia is reported to be very rare among primitives who stay on their ancestral diets.

The Importance of Chromium

There's a *chromium* content in bran, too. Chromium is used by the body to create a "glucose-tolerance factor" that we need to help us avoid or mitigate diabetes. Since diabetes is meaningfully associated with susceptibility to heart disease, atherosclerosis, and cancer, sources of chromium obviously should be protected. But they aren't. Sugar, like flour, has lost its chromium, and we have observed that the incidence of diabetes increases in rural Africans as they raise their sugar intake.

Samples of tissue from the bodies of people killed by heart attacks are usually low in chromium. While Americans tend to be low in it—the more so as they grow older—Africans' tissues contain a good bit of it, particularly in those areas where both diabetes and heart disease are very rare. When chromium deficiency is induced in animals, the blood vessels begin to accumulate the fatty deposits associated with heart attacks in human beings.

11. How'd You Like to Be a Pig?

There was once a song that plaintively inquired, "How'd you like to be a pig?" From the standpoint of good diet for good health, it's a proposition worth entertaining. As I pointed out earlier, we feed pigs superbly on what is removed from the white flour used to make our bran-less, fiber-deficient simulacrum of bread—the bread that Jean Mayer, of Harvard, has remarked would not be accepted as bread in his native France. (I don't know why, since French bread today has the same lack of fiber and nutrients as ours.) At any rate, *we* eat the bread, the white-flour products, and the overprocessed cereals, and the pigs subsist on the residues of the grain. As a result, the animal's diet shows these superiorities to white flour:

> 21 times the vitamin B_1
> 14 times the vitamin B_2
> 16 times the niacin
> 14 times the vitamin B_6
> 4 times the pantothenic acid
> 11 times the folic acid
> 17 times the vitamin E

   2 times the choline
   7 times the calcium
   9 times the phosphorus
12 times the magnesium
12 times the potassium
   3 times the sodium
   2 times the chromium
14 times the manganese
   6 times the iron
42 times the cobalt
   7 times the copper
12 times the zinc
   3 times the molybdenum

Dr. Henry Schroeder of Dartmouth, an authority on mineral metabolism, cited the above as evidence that white bread contributes calories without supplying the agents to put those calories to work properly in the body.

Many of the nutrients the body requires are supplied naturally by bran. Others are supplied by the germ of the grain, which joins bran in the white-flour residues fed to pigs instead of people. Africans enjoy the benefits of both germ and bran, for their carbohydrates escape the rolling mills.

It is at this point in a classroom lecture that one of my university students will arise to announce that 6 per cent of the public *do* buy whole-wheat bread. This statistic is particularly discouraging to me after I have spent decades trying to wean the public away from bubble-gum-and-balloon breads. It is equally discouraging to my students when they realize that even whole-wheat bread doesn't necessarily convey all the nutritional values of the entire wheat seed—that a significant part of the bran may have found its way to pig feed even when the label accurately describes the loaf as "100 per cent whole wheat" or as made from "stone-ground flour."

These remarks may jar even those who consider themselves nutritionally sophisticated. Let me explain that the fiber in grains is really a protective outer coating. Since it's external, very little milling will remove very substantial proportions of it—and milled it must be if the seed is to be converted into flour. In fact, so much of the fiber is removed in the earliest stages of grinding the wheat seeds into flour that further processing—even to the extreme needed to achieve white flour—only raises the depletion of fiber by a relatively small 9 per cent. This is not an argument in favor of shrugging one's shoulders and choosing bread by punching it to ascertain if the arm will disappear in it up to the elbow. The whole-grain loaf is still better nutrition. But this does explain the emphasis in high-fiber diets on the use of bran itself as a supplement.

Vegetarians will be quick to remind us that fiber is also provided by fruits and vegetables. It definitely is, but it's a different type; it's also from a much more expensive source, and it isn't as effective as bran.* Then, too, there are obviously limits to the amount of fruit one can or should eat, for too much sugar, from whatever source, is still undesirable; and there are limits to the quantities of vegetables the average person is willing to consume. (Such a limitation exists for some people with bread and baked products, too, of course.) For these reasons, the addition of bran as a supplement provides the most feasible way of restoring a useful type and amount of fiber to your diet.

Bread

For those who thrive on high-carbohydrate diets, I recommend baking your own nutritious, high-fiber bread based on whole-grain flour ground fresh in your own mill. There are small mills for home use; though many of them are unfortunately quite costly, they are certainly much cheaper than the medical bills for diverticulosis, rectal polyps, or bowel cancer. Making your own flour allows you to capitalize on the overall high nutritional values of fresh flour, and if you bake your own bread you can add extra bran to your recipe—up to 10 per cent—and thus maximize the amount of fiber your bread will contain.

---

* The fiber of carrots, however, has a particularly desirable effect.

Dr. Thomas L. Cleave, who pioneered the research with bran, argues compellingly for the use of both whole-grain bread *and* a bran supplement. This is *not* the doctrine of "If a little is good, more is better." He is concerned with compensating for the removal of fiber from sugar, for this is a loss even more drastic than the loss that occurs in the milling of flour. And with sugar supplying up to 25 per cent of the calories in millions of "civilized" diets, it's obvious that restoration of fiber to bread alone still leaves a gap in the dietary supply.

Cleave remarks: "In anyone taking a true whole-meal flour, the need for taking unprocessed bran is roughly proportional to his or her consumption of (refined) sugar." Since *all* sugar—white, yellow, brown, and raw—is refined, a bran supplement is not only a must for those who eat white flour and desirable for those who eat whole grains, but is *mandatory* for those who use sugar as a major food, rather than in limited quantities as a condiment (which is sugar's proper role).

12. Sugar Bowls, "Hidden" Sugar, and Common Sense

Nobody will admit to eating preposterous amounts of sugar, though we manufacture and import more than one hundred pounds per person per year. And the average person thinks of his sugar consumption in terms of the sugar bowl, but the hidden sugar in the diet is the real troublemaker.

There is sugar in tomato ketchup. There are five teaspoonfuls of sugar in a doughnut, and more if it's glazed. A portion of apple pie supplies twelve teaspoons of sugar—eighteen if you take it with ice cream, as many people do. (Ice cream itself is 16 per cent sugar.) A slice of cherry pie contains fourteen teaspoons of sugar. A piece of gum yields half a teaspoonful. There is likely to be sugar in the antacid you take to offset the indigestion you started by eating too much sugar. There is even sugar in salt: you'll find dextrose listed on the label.

Incessant and insensate abuse of the sweetener creates deficiencies in vitamin B complex, the need for which is *raised* by sugar intake.

And even as this is happening to our bodies, sugar processors are selling bagasse as fuel and as a base for wallboard. Bagasse is the fiber removed from the sweetener. The basis for Cleave's concern about the intake of refined sugar, previously noted, becomes clear, does it not?

Apart from its lack of fiber and the vitamins and minerals we need to metabolize it, sugar is reported to cause unfavorable changes in the bacterial flora of the bowel. In addition, sugar has been accused by Dr. John Yudkin, physician-biochemist, of raising the content of insulin, triglycerides, and uric acid in the blood; of increasing free fatty acids at the aorta; of boosting the stomach's hydrochloric-acid and pepsin levels; of increasing the adhesiveness of blood platelets; and of shrinking the pancreas, exponentially enlarging the liver, and enlarging the adrenal glands. And sugar assuredly places stress on the body, prodding it in the direction of diabetes, hypoglycemia (low blood sugar), strokes, heart attacks, and gastric ulcer.

Obviously, sugar intake must be reduced if you wish to fully capitalize upon the protection of a high-fiber diet. Your bran intake must be adjusted to compensate not only for the loss of bran in the milling of flour, but for the amount of sugar in your diet as well. (No one can succeed in getting rid of sugar entirely, for it is naturally present in many foods, and it is added to thousands more.)

Cutting Down on Sugar

Before we discuss bran dosage and means of incorporating it in your recipes and meals, let's spend a few minutes in helping you cut down on sugar intake. If you taste your beverages before you sweeten them, you'll find they really require less sweetening than you've been doing. Lemon tastes better on melon than sugar. Canned fruits packed *without* sugar syrup taste more like fresh fruits. The amount of sugar specified in many cookbook recipes can be reduced. (This should be done gradually. Don't try eliminating all sugar in recipes, for you will discover some—particularly in baking—in which at least *some* sugar is needed for acceptable texture.) And if you bring your protein intake nearer to the ideal with more emphasis on meat, fish, fowl, cheese, eggs, legumes, and nuts, you will usually reduce your craving for sweets.

What About Artificial Sweeteners?

We are not proposing that you reduce your intake of sugar, a dangerous and overused food, by raising your intake of the synthetic sweeteners that are currently under scrutiny. The objective is to retrain your palate. The evidence for and against cyclamates and saccharine is so mixed that no one can make more than an educated guess about the advisability of using them. The molecules of these chemicals are small and have a way of penetrating cells they shouldn't enter. If you are going to use them, do so in moderation. Do not abuse them as you have sugar, and stop using them entirely every third week to let the body excrete the residues.

Reduction of sugar intake calls for nothing more than common sense. A tart apple pie is less cloying to the palate than one laden with sugar. You don't spoon sugar over fresh fruit—why buy canned fruit in heavy syrup? (If you refuse to consume the water-packed variety, at least opt for light syrup and discard most of it before you eat the fruit.) Honey, which differs not at all from sugar in its impact on the body, offers one advantage: it is sweeter than sugar, and you're likely to use less. Apply common sense to desserts, too. It doesn't make sense to buy flavored gelatin desserts, whether sweetened with sugar or with artificial sweeteners, for they are a hodgepodge of artificial flavor and coal-tar dyes. Buy whole gelatin, and make your own gelatin desserts. By doing so you escape the 85-per-cent-sugar-15-per-cent-gelatin formula of the commercial varieties.

Most of the dry breakfast cereals contain

significant amounts of added sugar, but, ironically, the chief offenders are among the group of "natural" cereals that are now sold in grocery stores and supermarkets. Some of these, unbelievably, may contain 30 per cent to 40 per cent sugar. If the word "sugar" occurs high on the list of ingredients on the label, it's a tip-off that the cereal will *not* supply enough fiber to offset the amount of sugar incorporated in it.

The following chart will be useful in helping you identify the foods which are richest in unwanted sugar.

Approximate Refined-Carbohydrate Content of Popular Foods

Expressed in Amounts Equivalent to Teaspoonsful of Sugar

100 grams = 20 teaspoonsful = 3½ ounces = 400 calories

Food	Amount	Serving	Sugar Equivalent
CANDY			
Hershey bar	60 gm.	10¢ size	7 tsp.
Chocolate cream	13 gm.	1 (35 to lb.)	2 tsp.
Chocolate fudge	30 gm.	1, 1½ inches sq. (15 to 1 lb.)	4 tsp.
Chewing gum		1 stick	⅓ tsp.
Life-saver		1 usual size	⅓ tsp.
CAKE			
Chocolate cake	100 gm.	2-layer with icing; 1/12 cake	15 tsp.
Angel cake	45 gm.	1/12 large cake	6 tsp.
Sponge cake	50 gm.	1/10 of average cake	6 tsp.
Cream puff (iced)	80 gm.	1 average, custard-filled	5 tsp.
Doughnut, plain	40 gm.	1, 3 inches in diameter	4 tsp.
COOKIES			
Macaroons	25 gm.	1 large or 2 small	3 tsp.

Gingersnaps	1 medium	6 gm.	1 tsp.
Brownies	1, 2 inches sq., ¾ inches thick	20 gm.	3 tsp.
CUSTARDS			
Custard, baked	½ cup		4 tsp.
Gelatin	½ cup		4 tsp.
Junket	⅛ quart		3 tsp.
ICE CREAM			
Ice cream	⅛ quart		5 to 6 tsp.
Water ice	⅛ quart		6 to 8 tsp.
PIE			
Apple pie	1/6 of med. pie		12 tsp.
Cherry pie	1/6 of med. pie		14 tsp.
Custard, coconut pie	1/6 of med. pie		10 tsp.
Pumpkin pie	1/6 of med. pie		10 tsp.
SAUCE			
Chocolate	1 heaping tsp.	30 gm.	4½ tsp.
Marshmallow	1 aver. serving (60 to 16 oz.)	7.6 gm.	1½ tsp.
SPREADS			
Jam	1 level tbsp. or 1 heaping tsp.	20 gm.	3 tsp.

81

Food	Amount	Serving	Sugar Equiv- alent
Jelly	20 gm.	1 level tbsp. or 1 heaping tsp.	2½ tsp.
Marmalade	20 gm.	1 level tbsp. or 1 heaping tsp.	3 tsp.
Honey	20 gm.	1 level tbsp. or 1 heaping tsp.	3 tsp.
MILK DRINKS			
Chocolate (all milk)		1 cup, 5 oz. milk	6 tsp.
Cocoa (all milk)		1 cup, 5 oz. milk	4 tsp.
Cocomalt (all milk)		1 glass, 8 oz. milk	4 tsp.
SOFT DRINKS			
Coca-Cola	180 gm.	1 bottle (6 oz.)	4⅓ tsp.
Ginger ale	180 gm.	6 oz. glass	4⅓ tsp.
COOKED FRUITS			
Peaches, canned in syrup	10 gm.	2 halves, 1 tbsp. juice	3½ tsp.
Rhubarb, stewed	100 gm.	½ cup sweetened	8 tsp.
Applesauce (no added sugar)	100 gm.	scant ½ cup	2 tsp.
Prunes, stewed, sweetened	100 gm.	4 to 5 med., 2 tbsp. juice	8 tsp.

82

DRIED FRUITS

Apricots	4 to 6 halves	30 gm.	4 tsp.
Prunes	3 to 4 medium	30 gm.	4 tsp.
Dates	3 to 4 stoned	30 gm.	4½ tsp.
Figs	1½ to 2 small	30 gm.	4 tsp.
Raisins	¼ cup	30 gm.	4 tsp.

FRUITS AND FRUIT JUICES

Fruit cocktail	½ cup, scant	120 gm.	5 tsp.
Orange juice	½ cup, scant	100 gm.	2 tsp.
Grapefruit juice, unsweetened	½ cup, scant	100 gm.	2-1/5 tsp.
Grape juice, commercial	½ cup, scant	100 gm.	3-2/3 tsp.
Pineapple juice, unsweetened	½ cup, scant	100 gm.	2-3/5 tsp.

13. A Bran Program:
Individual Tolerances, How and How Much, What Kind, When and Where—and Yogurt

Before I outline a bran-intake schedule for adults and children, let's consider the mythical Mrs. McCann who can eat no bran—or, at least, very little of it. Contrary to past nutritional beliefs, her type is rare, and most people will tolerate bran very well—even those with irritable intestinal tracts.

To buttress that last point, we can turn to the *British Medical Journal*, where we find Dr. N. S. Painter and other physicians making a statement echoed by many doctors: "A trial lasting for four years of a high-residue low-sugar diet given to seventy patients with diverticular disease (colon) was 85 per cent effective in relieving or reducing symptoms." In spite of the explicitness of this finding, those with such digestive disorders should *not* experiment on their own. If you have a serious disorder, you need medical supervision.

As a member of an average American family, you have probably been eating a low-fiber diet since your first spoonful of baby food. (Many baby foods, *some of which should not be,* are low in fiber residue.) This means that you've been on a low-fiber intake for years. The fact that you're free of symptoms is meaningless, for the incubation period for the diseases caused by lack of fiber is very long. Therefore, bran supplements are useful for those who are not yet troubled and don't want to be, as well as for those who already have chronic constipation.

Coarsely ground bran is sometimes, but not always, more effective and tolerance to finely ground bran is sometimes better. Do *not* buy costly name-brand fiber mixtures in the health-food stores. They are represented as being superior to bran and some of them are (you can use some in smaller doses), but when they sell at $4.95 per pound, you might as well stick with bran. The smaller doses of the name-brand mixes of ground psyllium, bran, carrot, cabbage, and the like may be significantly helpful when active colon disease is present and intolerance to bran forces reduction of the bran dose to an ineffective level. But that's likely to be a rare situation. One teaspoonful of finely ground bran daily can effectively normalize elimination and stool-transit time. I have known this to be the case even with an individual suffering from diverticular disease and chronic constipation, and it occurred totally without disturbing effects.

Large bran tablets are now appearing on health-food stores' shelves. For some people, these may prove a convenience. But a considerable number of them will be needed daily when maximum doses of fiber are necessary, and, for those with very inefficient digestive function, any hard-pressed tablet may present a problem —it may be excreted intact, with no evidence that the body has managed to utilize any part of the content. (This applies not only to bran but to many other preparations in tablet form, including vitamins and minerals, which explains the advantages of liquid vitamin-and-mineral supplements—particularly for older people.) However, if you have no difficulty in breaking down tablets and your life-style demands a "gulp-and-gallop" kind of nutrition, such bran tablets will be useful and convenient.

Cereals

I take a dim view of the prepared, ready-to-eat bran cereals that are available in flake form, sometimes combined with raisins. This dim view is based on my indignation at the cereal companies' selling us the bran they have removed from their other products, and on the heat treatment to which such cereals are inevitably subjected. *It is raw bran we are looking for.*

A single serving of a bran cereal will fall far short of supplying the amount of fiber many individuals require if they are to profit fully by this change in dietary habits. And some bran cereals contain artificial preservatives, particularly BHA and BHT. These are anti-oxidants, originally formulated to preserve the colors in *motion-picture film!* Adverse effects have been reported for both—skin cancer has occurred after local application of BHA; changes in brain function have been seen in animals fed BHT.

I have always regarded as incompetent any program for human diet that generalizes about human nutritional needs and dietetic tolerances. This is the fallacy in the "recommended dietary allowances" set by the F.D.A. for vitamins and other nutrients. One might as well propose to bring prices of bras, shoes, and false teeth down by making them all in one size! Humans' biochemical differences are so great that a bloodhound can pick one suspect out of a thousand because no two of us even smell alike. We have differences in our needs and tolerances for fiber, too.

Those who respond nobly to a single teaspoonful of fine bran daily are probably outnumbered by those who need two or three table-spoonfuls daily. There are those who profit from taking very finely milled bran but cannot tolerate coarsely ground bran in the same quantity. And about one-third of those suffering from irritable bowel syndrome or diverticular disease will not be able to tolerate—much less profit by—*any* type or amount of bran. The rest benefit, but optimal doses are highly individual. Generally speaking—insofar as generalization is possible—*those who have had no difficulties with whole-grain breads and cereals and with salads will find bran acceptable.*

Because of individual differences in needs and tolerances, I raise fiber intake slowly, beginning with *a teaspoonful at breakfast.* This is gradually raised to *three teaspoons* a day—divided among meals and snacks. If the hoped-for result (which I'll describe) does not happen, the dose is raised to *two teaspoonfuls* at each meal, for a total of six per day. That is not the ceiling, for there are individuals who require three tablespoons of bran a day to achieve maximum benefits. Young children will, of course, need less. Children under six need perhaps a half teaspoonful per day; from age six to puberty, about a half teaspoonful three times daily.

In the early days of a bran-supplement program, there is an increase in the amount of flatulence—gas that is passed. This gas *must* be passed. When gas is not permitted to exit and is returned to the bowel, the natural order of matters is being reversed, and great physical pressure may be brought upon the colon. There are physicians who regard gas retention as one of the more common ways of worsening, or even starting, diverticular disease.

As one goes along with the bran program, the stool should lose much of its odor, for the bacteria are now being thwarted in their attack on the stool because it is moving through the bowel faster. The movement should be large and should be passed without any effort. (This is important, for straining is one of the causes of varicose veins and hemorrhoids.)

The best vehicle for bran is a good cereal. It is obviously irrational to add it to an over-processed one that is deprived of its own fiber and laden with additives—that is, almost any cereal in the supermarket. In my experience, oatmeal is a good vehicle. When you're using it, remember that large amounts of sugar will defeat your purpose in adding the bran—at least in part. Thus, buy oatmeal that has had a minimum of sugar added by the manufacturer.

Some people take bran in fruit juices; some add it to applesauce. (Applesauce packed without added sugar is now available.) Suggestions like these provide the breakfast vehicle for bran.

A Total Program

If you decide to adopt my total program, you will be using yogurt, lactic-acid yeast, or tablets of the "friendly" lactobacillus organisms. That means that yogurt will be a logical vehicle for bran, and it proves to be a good one. Contrary to the advice I've seen in medical articles on this subject, flavored yogurt should *not* be used. The quantity of sugar in some of these products is beyond believing (there are more calories from sugar than from yogurt in some of them). Vanilla yogurt, free of the sugar-saturated fruit preserves in many of the flavored products, might seem preferable, but it often contains more sugar than most of the other varieties. *Buy plain yogurt, or, better yet, make your own.*

A simple and inexpensive home yogurt incubator is available; it's just a hot plate with recesses for jars that holds the temperature to the one favorable for growing yogurt cultures. The homemade product will cost you much less than the commercial one, and you can add fresh fruit to plain yogurt—or, if you want a sweet taste without added sugar, use real vanilla in your yogurt. A teaspoonful of bran per cup of yogurt is a palatable blend.

If you bake at home, add 10 per cent bran to whole-wheat bread recipes. Two slices of bread will provide a sizeable percentage of the day's ration of fiber, and this may constitute the evening meal's contribution to your bran intake. Bran muffins for snacks are another alternative.

When you're not in a position to adopt any of these suggestions at a given meal or snack period, bran tablets can be used to provide the fiber quotient for at least one meal or snack. Other recipe suggestions are given in Chapter 21.

14. Bran and Heart Disease: Some Pros and Cons

There is no doubt that ischemic heart disease—the attacks of coronary thrombosis that kill millions in the western world—simply does not occur in the Africans whose diets were studied and found to be rich in unprocessed carbohydrates. Unprocessed carbohydrates are high in fiber. But heart disease is also rare with *other* Africans whose diets are *not* rich in cereal fiber. And heart attacks are largely unknown among those whose diets are *low* in fats and cholesterol, but there are also groups whose diets are *high* in cholesterol and fat among whom heart attacks are almost unheard of.

To those content with simple explanations of complex phenomena, the immunity of the fiber-eaters is explained by an unexpected effect of bran—it increases the excretion of cholesterol. But to accept that, one has to be persuaded that excess cholesterol is in fact *the* cause of hardening of the arteries and associated heart disease. And then what does one do to explain those Africans whose diet is low in cereal fiber and high in cholesterol—and who are still innocent of heart disease?

I submit that there is a basic requirement for accepting the hypothesis that bran, by promoting excretion of cholesterol, will wipe out cardiac disease: one must be scientifically a little naïve, and not too familiar with the difficulties of unraveling the interlocking actions of nutrients in the human body. If bran is a broom that sweeps excess cholesterol from the body and thereby prevents heart attacks, then the American lack of fiber in the diet should cause heart disease in both sexes in the same frequency; and this it does not do. Men are much more susceptible to heart attack than premenopausal women—and there is no basis for a theory that women, before menopause, eat more fiber than men, and then, after the event, suddenly reduce their intake.

This simplistic "solution" to the complex problem of heart disease and nutrition reminds me of an old story. A man drinks whiskey and soda on Monday, followed by gin and soda on Tuesday, topped off with vodka and soda on Wednesday. Since he is ineffably drunk on all three occasions, this is scientific proof that soda is intoxicating!

To view cholesterol objectively, one must evaluate the helpfulness of bran in increasing excretion of cholesterol. Nature didn't invent cholesterol to provide cardiologists with an annuity, but as a basis for the manufacture of sex (and other) hormones and of bile salts, without which digestion of fats would be impossible. Cholesterol is also essential in the creation of the "insulation" (myelin sheaths) that keeps our nerves from short-circuiting. Those intent on banishing all high-cholesterol foods from the diet—even from the diet of newborn infants—seem to ignore the indispensability of the substance.

And then there's the fact that nature has provided the body with the capacity to manufacture the majority of the cholesterol it needs. Cholesterol supply, then, could *increase* in some individuals when the dietary supply is reduced! This, of course, could make a restricted diet an exercise in futility.

Those who play the game with cholesterol blood levels in which the prizes go to those who achieve the lowest possible figures are sometimes guilty of ignoring other factors in the blood. The triglycerides, phospholipids, and high density lipoproteins are regarded by many nutritionists as being at least as significant in atherosclerosis and heart attacks as is cholesterol. And "blood levels" of cholesterol, triglycerides, etc., simply indicate how the bodily processes are doing—whether they're normal or "out of whack."

Consider a nutritionist's concern with abnormally elevated blood triglycerides. To him, this is but a symptom reflecting abnormally high intake of sugar or impaired tolerance for it or both. Sugar tolerance can be tested, and, if necessary, improved. (People can be taught to recognize that they consume vast amounts of sugar from unsuspected sources.) The important point: Taking steps to lower elevated blood triglycerides may mean the patient will avoid a heart attack caused by hardening of the arteries—and "cholesterol" hasn't even been considered.

This brings up another important point. Those who attribute to bran the Africans' freedom from heart attacks have sometimes failed to consider that these people also enjoy the benefits of a diet rich in vitamins and minerals, and almost totally lacking in overconcentrated sugar. The evidence from Africa also suggests that those who try to persuade us that animal fats grease the slide into eternity are *wrong*.

At least the bran approach doesn't force you to exclude foods that contain cholesterol from your diet. This is certainly a good thing, for, by coincidence, foods that are high in cholesterol are also highest in overall nutritional values—eggs, liver and other organ meats, milk and many dairy products.

Unsaturated fats are highly recommended in nutrition. Researchers are already commenting caustically on the dividends we're *not* receiving from raising our intake of vegetable oils (unsaturated fats), for the incidence of heart attacks has certainly not yielded to that dietary trend. Of course, there *are* still pediatricians who place babies on low-fat formula, indicating that they believe nature created a poor food when she invented breast milk; and there are still medical men who recommend diets that attempt to avoid *all* foods containing cholesterol. This would be the logical time to note that man has consumed both fats and cholesterol throughout his millennia-long career as a huntsman-herder. The recent innovations in his diet are sugar and overprocessed grains, cereals, and flour, not fats and cholesterol.

15. The Many Ways to a Healthy Heart

Simple logic will tell anyone that the "cause" of a phenomenon can't be the cause when the phenomenon occurs in its absence. The opposite, of course, is also true: When the "cause" is present and the result doesn't materialize, the "cause" can't be the cause.

We must now consider some pointed questions. Are there people with normal or even low blood cholesterol who *do* have heart attacks? Of course. Are there people with elevated blood cholesterol who *don't* get heart attacks? Of course. Are there those who eat large quantities of high-cholesterol, high-animal-fat foods, and suffer no cardiac penalties—even when they consume limited amounts of fiber? Yes. The Masai tribesmen in Africa are good examples of this—their diet is based on large amounts of meat, milk, and blood, and includes *some* vegetables and fruits. It certainly doesn't emphasize unprocessed carbohydrates, rich in bran. Yet these magnificent physical specimens have the same freedom from heart disease that, in other

African tribes, has confidently been attributed to the high cereal-fiber intake that promotes the excretion of cholesterol.

One theory to explain Masai immunity to cardiovascular disease postulates that an unknown protective factor is supplied by their fermented milk, which they drink in large quantities. Nobel Prize winner Ilya Ilyich Metchnikoff must be turning over in his grave! While we're mentioning this pioneer again—he's the man who attributed Bulgarians' excellent health and long life span to yogurt—let's remember that the proponents of today's low-cholesterol diet describe dairy products as life-shortening. This is a gross oversimplification of complex phenomena, and it is *not* a reasonable argument against using yogurt as part of the high-fiber diet.

At the height of the anti-cholesterol fad, attention was addressed to the Yemeni (Black Jews) who have migrated to Israel. They took with them to their new land a high immunity to diabetes and to coronary disease—and they gradually lost it during twenty-five years of residence in their new home. The rising incidence of the two diseases, which eventually climbed to the accustomed Israeli level, was immediately attributed to the immigrants' adoption of Israeli foods like butter, cream, and eggs, with their "lethal" content of cholesterol.

As a trustee of the International Academy of

Preventive Medicine, I was one of the hosts of Dr. A. M. Cohen, who studied the changes in the Yemeni diet. He showed that by far the greatest dietary innovation the Yemenites had made involved a sharp rise in sugar intake; there was little change in the amount of fat or cholesterol they consumed. Such studies are assiduously ignored by those who have adopted the low-cholesterol theory—and suffered sharp attacks of closing of the mind.

What About Water?

In the papers and books on the virtues of bran as a weapon against cardiac disease, I find no mention of the characteristics of the *water* consumed by Africans. Whether it is hard or soft water is more than an academic question. Repeated studies in many parts of the world show significantly fewer heart attacks in hard-water areas. In fact, there was even a study that was—by chance—controlled. The Florida city involved shifted from a soft-water city supply to hard-water wells—and a striking drop in the incidence of heart attacks resulted.

The hard-water phenomenon operates independently of blood cholesterol levels. Observations have shown that comparatively high average cholesterol levels among the citizens in hard-water cities have had no detrimental effect —the heart attack rate is still lower than in soft-water cities in which the citizens' cholesterol levels are lower.

I have discussed these observations with Henry Schroeder, an authority on the minerals, toxic and beneficial, in our environment, and he has indicated that it is difficult to decide whether hard water carries minerals that protect us, or soft water picks up undesirable amounts of toxic minerals from, say, the plumbing that conveys it to us.* When this question is settled—and, obviously, not until then—we may be able to fix the role, if any, of African water in determining the level of cardiac integrity. And until that question of water (among others) is settled, eulogies of bran as *sure* prevention for heart attacks simply aren't scientifically justified.

In fact, until the whole cholesterol debate is resolved, no definitive statements about heart disease and bran or any other dietary factor will be tenable. Consider, for instance, the studies undertaken by the American Cancer Society, which reviewed the cases of 804,409 persons with no previous history of heart disease or stroke. The society scrutinized the diets of

---

* Schroeder has also pointed out that the cadmium in our environment threatens us with high blood pressure, which is, of course, a factor in heart attacks. The antidote for cadmium is zinc. Ironically, when wheat is made into our highly processed white flour it loses much of its zinc but retains most of its cadmium. On the other hand, the unprocessed carbohydrates of rural Africans have a fairly favorable zinc-cadmium ratio. Note, incidentally, that this factor in heart attack has nothing to do with cholesterol.

14,819 of these people who died from heart disease and 4,099 who died from stroke within a six-year period. Among the dead, they identified those who had eaten substantial amounts of eggs and saturated fats—and those who ate few eggs (or none at all) and ate little meat and few fried foods or avoided them altogether. Conclusion: The death rate from heart disease and stroke was *lower* in those who ate eggs, higher among egg-avoiders. This observation, too, is ignored by those who are fascinated by the numbers game with blood cholesterol levels.

Michael DeBakey, the noted heart surgeon, has had the opportunity to inspect arteries more intimately than the vast majority of those who head the anti-cholesterol crusade. He has published a paper stating that he has *not* found a consistent, significant relationship between levels of blood cholesterol and the extent of atherosclerotic involvement of the blood-vessel walls.

What about the studies interpreted as *proving* that a low intake of cholesterol and animal fat reduces the incidence of heart attacks? In such research, there is an unavoidable, uncontrolled, and very significant variable. The majority of the subjects in such studies are, possibly for the first time in their lives, eating planned, carefully supervised, adequate diets. This naturally has a potent influence on well-being, but no attempt has been made to measure how great the influence is.

Vitamins and Minerals

A researcher at Johns Hopkins University has published several reports on his success in averting heart attacks by administering very small doses of vitamins and highly absorbable minerals. It is pertinent that many of the nutrients involved in this research are supplied *naturally* by bran and the germ of whole grains.

Then there are experts who posit that electrical disturbances in the natural pacemaker of the heart precede and, in some unknown way, precipitate heart attacks. The *Shute Bulletin,* published by the pioneering Shute Institute of Canada, cites the importance of vitamin B_{12} —richly supplied by the Masai high-protein diet —as a beneficial influence on the electrical activity of the heart. The effect of vitamin B_{12} is described as second only to the effect of vitamin E—the richest natural source of which is the germ of whole grains.

Much of the cholesterol-causes-heart-attacks theory loses momentum when the process of hardening of the arteries is minutely studied. The first invader of the artery wall *isn't* cholesterol, *isn't* a fat, but is a glycoprotein—a combination of sugar and protein. Another bit of folklore that may one day be retired from scientific circulation is that a clot, perhaps snagged on a lesion in a hardened coronary artery, shuts off part of the supply of blood feeding the heart muscle and invariably causes heart attack.

There are physiologists and cardiologists who believe—for good reasons—that the clot follows, rather than causes, the attack—is, in fact, *caused by* the attack. Another group are studying the dynamics of fluid behavior when the fluid contains clotting substances, is under physical pressure in a closed system, and must circulate around sharp bends and curves. This is, of course, a description of blood and its circulation, and the fluid-dynamics studies may find that atherosclerosis begins as a mechanical rather than a biochemical problem.

Other Factors

Some consideration must also be given to the kaleidoscopic interplay of other factors that affect cholesterol metabolism or have direct influence on cardiac health. The *thyroid gland,* for instance, plays a role in controlling the levels of blood fats, including cholesterol—in fact, it is so intimately involved with blood fats that cholesterol blood levels are sometimes used as a means of rechecking thyroid function when more direct tests of the gland give equivocal results.

The extent to which physical activity is involved in cardiac health is still undefined. Joggers on low-cholesterol diets will still, in some cases, suffer heart attacks. Personality traits have been blamed as well: Hard-driving, perfectionist personalities, struggling with constant deadlines, seem more vulnerable to cardiac disease, and so, in a recent analysis, do those individuals who use power as a substitute for love. And how do we deal with the possible influence of the severe emotional disturbances that so often precede heart attacks? Or with the role of genetics in determining circulatory reactions to a given diet—low in cholesterol or high, high in fiber or low?

I have written this section—in which I could have cited many other pertinent observations from scientific literature—because I am troubled by the attempt to make bran a panacea that will free mankind of ischemic heart disease.

While the scientific papers that document the action of bran against bowel cancer are voluminous and competently written, I have been able to find only *one* paper that proposes a role for bran in reducing the production of lithocolate. (Lithocolate is the abnormal product of normal bile salts that is said to discourage liver production of the salts.) This book will therefore make no claim that bran in the diet is an easy way to cardiac health. If cardiac health proves to be one of the many dividends of a high-fiber diet, we'll all be grateful.

16. The Nutrition-Packed Wheat Germ— Bran's Natural Companion

You're reading this book on the high-fiber diet, its contributions to immunities to many of our diseases, and what it can do for us. Suddenly, in this section, you're about to find yourself in the middle of a discussion of quasi-hormones, spontaneous abortion and other aspects of impaired reproductive efficiency, and why vitamin E isn't the middle letter in the word "sex." Don't wonder where you went off the track; if you'll be patient for a moment, you'll learn why this apparent detour takes you directly toward other dividends you receive from the good foods in a high-fiber diet.

Perhaps you'll recall the tragic case of the young women with vaginal cancer, induced before birth by the administration of diethylstilbestrol (DES) to their pregnant mothers. More than three hundred such cases of cancer have been identified so far, and there have been several deaths from it. This is a tragic illustration of disease caused by the physician's treatment. Males born of mothers who have taken DES have also paid a price—not in cancer, but in reduced masculinity.

The obstetricians of the 1950s who administered DES to expectant mothers had an urgent motive and the best of intentions. They were trying to avert threatened abortions. But the real tragedy of this medical error has never been mentioned in any of the many papers devoted to the histories of the young women who developed vaginal cancer. The fact is that the administration of the dangerous hormone wasn't necessary. Not only was it not the only remedy available for threatened abortion, but the obstetricians could have saved just as many of the pregnancies with a totally harmless nutritional treatment known since 1936 to promote fertility and to rescue jeopardized pregnancies in cows, goats, sheep—and human mothers. That treatment consists of an improved diet and the supplementing of it with high-quality wheat-germ oil.

This brings us to the point: The oil from the germ of the grain is one of the automatic dividends rural Africans receive when they eat the natural, unprocessed carbohydrates that also supply the bran in their high-fiber diets. The fiber alone can't be given credit for the superior health and reproductive efficiency of the unwesternized rural Africans.

Don't think this is academic. We of the western world, despite our record of population explosions, also have a record of dismal reproductive efficiency. Too many of our women can't conceive; too many of our men are infertile; too many of our pregnancies abort or are threatened by complications; too many of our babies are born deformed or unhealthy. And the germ oil we so nonchalantly remove from our white flour and processed grains and cereals has been helpful in the prevention and the treatment of many of the tendencies to reproductive failure. (Incidentally, the helpful action of the germ oil does *not* come from its vitamin E content, despite the tenacity of this widely held belief.)

At the University of Illinois, Professor Thomas Cureton investigated the properties of a neuromuscular agent drawn from wheat-germ oil by my good friend Dr. Ezra Levin, a microbiologist. That substance, known to nutritionists as *octacosanol*—and to the chemist as a 27-carbon, straight chain, waxy alcohol—proved remarkably effective in rehabilitating flabby, underexercised, middle-aged men Given supplements of wheat-germ oil in concentrated form, plus a program of exercise patterned to their needs and tolerances. the men responded by turning back the physiological clock. Physical endurance and heart performance improved to a significant degree. (It is interesting to note that the study group also included trained athletes, who also benefited.)

Despite this monumental research at the University of Illinois, confirmed in both doctoral and master's theses, dieticians still make dogmatic statements that *no* food supplement has any effect on muscular performance or athletic ability. But then, there are dieticians who say there is no significant difference between whole-wheat and white bread, whole-grain and white flour, brown rice and white rice—ad infinitum, ad nauseam.

During years of research in muscular dystrophy at the Payne Whitney Clinic in New York, a neurologist administered the octacosanol concentrate to some patients—with resulting benefit. In my function as a consultant in nutrition, I have often been responsible for physicians' administration of this wheat-germ-oil agent in the treatment of multiple sclerosis, muscular atrophy, myasthenia gravis, amyotonia congenita, several types of cerebral palsy, brain damage, post-stroke syndrome, myositis, dermatomyositis, and numerous other disorders of nerve-muscle function.

With such ailments the medical armament is often limited—and, more often, of limited value. The germ-oil agent isn't a panacea. But among those who read this book I am sure there will be some who, thanks to octacosanol, are today socially and vocationally functioning when a few years ago they were crippled with multiple sclerosis or other nerve-muscle disorders.

Therapeutic responses to nutritional factors always imply the possibility that an opportunity for prophylaxis has been lost. Translation: When a sick person responds to concentrated wheat-germ oil, should we not wonder whether his life history of eating white bread and other degerminated cereals was the prelude to his illness? Whether the Africans' diet, with its undegerminated grains, might not have averted or mitigated the disorder?

Prostaglandins

High school students will tell you that our hormones are manufactured by our glands. Some endocrinologists long ago disagreed with this concept, for there is some evidence that *every organ in the body makes its own hormones*. That theory was strengthened with the discovery of hormone-like factors, the *prostaglandins*, hailed as the medical discovery of the age. Almost every *cell* in the body produces prostaglandins.

There are many kinds of prostaglandins acting in many ways, and many have conflicting effects. There are prostaglandins that improve circulation, lower blood pressure, reduce stomach-acid production, and promote very rapid healing in duodenal ulcer patients. There are others that ease muscle contractions during birth, thus shutting off the flow of blood in the umbilical cord (so that when animals sever it they are not threatened with hemorrhage). There are prostaglandins that bring on the menstrual flow—these offer great hope of a harmless method of birth-control, and of safe, easy abortions in the fourth to sixth months of pregnancy; it may also develop that prostaglandins can be used to prevent the clots which cause strokes. This is only a partial list of types of prostaglandins. A fascinating aspect of their chemistry is that at least thirteen of them so far identified are based on a fat called *arachidonic acid*. This is synthesized by the body from another fat, which is richly and primarily supplied by the oil in the germ of grains—such as wheat germ.

Neither arachidonic acid nor its precursor comes to you in useful amounts from dietary sources other than the germ of grains. This places great emphasis on the nutritional contributions of nuts, seeds, and whole grains (which are, of course, seeds).

The roll call of benefits from wheat and other grain germs is still far from complete. Wheat germ supplies phytosterol and sitosterol, which reduce cholesterol absorption and concentration in the blood. These are points to be remembered by those who eulogize bran as if *it alone* were the significant variable in whole-grain versus overprocessed carbohydrates. It happens that wheat germ, in addition to giving you the benefits I've just been talking about, is a good source of fiber and is a fine, staple food source of B-complex vitamins and trace minerals, and the *best* natural cereal source of vitamin E.

Using Wheat Germ in Your Diet

What you have read in this section is part of the scientific justification for a deliberate effort to restore grain germs—particularly wheat germ—to your diet. Note that you can profit not only by the intake of the whole grains, but by adding wheat germ itself to your recipes and menus.

The simplest way to use wheat germ is as a cereal, with your bran added to it. In lieu of this, wheat germ can be added to (good) cereals. If you bake with white flour (which should be unbleached—bleaching destroys vitamin E) or whole-wheat flour, you can routinely incorporate in the recipe a teaspoonful of wheat germ to each cup of flour. This ordinarily doesn't call for any readjustment of the proportions of other ingredients, nor will it be detectable in the average baked product—it will just make things taste better. When larger percentages of wheat germ are used, it is often necessary to reduce the shortening in the recipe slightly (wheat germ contains oil) and to increase the liquid.

Don't do what most converts to good nutrition do—go overboard. Wheat germ is very high in good quality protein. Using excessive amounts of it will yield cakes, cookies, and bread that will have to be carried to the table by strong men.

I am often asked if toasted wheat germ has lost much value. The losses I have measured are not significant, and some people who refuse to eat the raw germ will accept the toasted variety. My nutritional preference, though, is for unprocessed and unheated wheat germ,* just as I prefer the equivalent in bran.

Don't buy wheat germ in paper bags or unsealed boxes. Like all good foods, it is highly perishable. Wheat germ in a vacuum-packed bottle is best; keep it in the refrigerator after it has been opened. *Don't* buy brands mixed with honey or other forms of sugar.

Be adventuresome in trying new recipes for wheat germ, for it will prove palatable in unexpected company. Example: Sauté onions in butter or margarine, add noodle-thin strips of liver —any kind of liver—and when the meat is cooked, which takes only a couple of minutes, sprinkle a little wheat germ on it. Then serve. You may be flabbergasted by calls for "seconds" with an organ meat!

Wheat-germ oil can be used as a supplement

* For full benefit, use wheat germ that has *not* been defatted, as many commercial brands have been.

—take a teaspoonful daily, or ten six-minim capsules. Or add wheat-germ oil to salad oil, fifty-fifty. (Its taste is a bit strong when it's used alone in a salad dressing.) Just don't cook with it—the manufacturers go to great pains not to expose this oil to excessive heat.

As you learn to use wheat germ, remember the dividends you are receiving—additional useful fiber, vitamin B complex, vitamin E, octocosanol, phytosterol, protein, sitosterol, and trace minerals. That list is not complete, but it does emphasize the importance of using bran's natural companion—the nutrition-packed germ.

17. For Women Only

Women may earn special dividends from the high-fiber diet and the BAMBY plan—they may gain increased resistance to breast cancer and a sharp reduction in symptoms associated with the menstrual cycle. This statement does not imply that a high-fiber diet will do less, overall, for a man's health; it merely indicates that women have some biological characteristics not shared by men. And it invites no confrontation with Women's Lib—it simply attempts to explore a subject that, like so many others in nutrition, is both poorly understood and a focal point for controversy.

After many years of research into dietary needs that are peculiar to women (in degree, if not in kind) because of their endocrine singularities, I am satisfied that optimal nutrition will in fact significantly lower susceptibility to cancer of the breast—and possibly to cancer of the uterus as well. By happy coincidence, the high-fiber diet, particularly when it is part of the BAMBY plan, supplies generous amounts of the nutrients that are critically important to women.

Synthetic Hormones

Estrogenic hormones are intimately involved here. You know that these hormones are ingredients in many birth-control pills, and that menopausal women are treated with estrogens. You have read articles concerning the occurrence of vaginal cancer in girls whose mothers, in pregnancy, were given a *synthetic* female hormone, diethylstilbestrol (DES). You may know that DES is used to speed weight gain in cattle, much to my distress and the distress of many other nutritionists.

Few women realize that the estrogens produced by their own ovaries may be as hazardous as a synthetic hormone like DES, and still fewer realize that some women produce five times as many hormones as other women do. Those who produce large amounts of estrogen may be in more danger of getting estrogen-dependent cancer *if* this hormone does, as many authorities believe, contribute to the disease. Thus such women may—unknowingly—be running a considerable risk of getting cancer of the breast and uterus, for these are estrogen-sensitive tissues.

One of the standard procedures in the effort to slow up the progress of breast cancer is to remove the ovaries. Although drastic, this is one way of relieving the breasts—and the tumor—

of the stimulation of estrogen. The operation was formerly done empirically—that is, without the physician's being sure it would do any good —for physicians could not predict which cancers would respond and which would not. Recently, though, a technique has been developed to identify *estrogen receptors* in the cancerous tissue. If such receptors are present, it means that the growth is dependent on estrogen, and that, in turn, promises that lowering the level of estrogen in the body—by removing the ovaries—will slow or even stop the growth of the cancer. There have been, in fact, rare cases where removal of the ovaries actually caused cancer of the breast to disappear.

There are many physicians who regard doses of estrogen for anyone but menopausal women as a kind of mindless Russian roulette. They don't object to supplementing the declining output of estrogen in menopausal and postmenopausal women, but they draw the line at giving doses of estrogen to younger women whose bodies are still busily manufacturing the hormone. There are, nonetheless, other practitioners who prescribe estrogen freely. The F.D.A. and drug manufacturers advise that these hormones must *not* be prescribed for women with latent cancer. But since "latent" in this sense means "concealed," how could a physician know if a female patient had "latent cancer"?

On the practice of giving estrogen, Dr. Roy Hertz of the National Cancer Institute remarked some years ago: "It is playing with fire. . . . We know that estrogens, when given in large doses over a prolonged period, will induce tumors of the breast, cervix, endometrium, pituitary, testicles, kidney, and bone marrow in mice, rats, rabbits, hamsters, and dogs. *These studies are applicable to man.*" It is of striking significance that the administration of *anti-estrogen* chemicals has been reported to cause shrinkage of cancers in more than 50 per cent of the women treated with them.

The Yin-Yang Principle

The human body is a biochemical-electrical phenomenon, maintaining a dynamic balance in the midst of forces of anarchy. The body operates on the Yin-Yang principle—for every force there is a counter-force; for every reaction, a counter-reaction; for every trigger, a safety mechanism that prevents the trigger from being pulled at the wrong time.

One would expect, then, that the marvelous organism we inhabit would in some way exercise braking actions on the activities of its glands. And that's exactly what it does. The system of controls on the glands involves the self-balancing feedback principle—for example, an excess level of thyroid hormone in the blood alerts the pituitary gland, which reacts by dampening production of a hormone that stimulates the thyroid.

In the case of estrogen, *two* means of control are exerted. One is the feedback principle, operating through the pituitary gland. The other control is exercised by the liver—with an important "if": *If the diet is adequate to support that function.*

A Vital Point

This brings us to a vital point of this chapter. It is perfectly possible to be well-fed by usual nutritional standards and yet to fail to supply the liver with optimal amounts of the nutrients it requires to help it control estrogen activity. This is a long way of saying that a "well-nourished" woman might earn many dividends if improvements in her diet encouraged the liver to control the production of estrogen more efficiently.

It seems more reasonable to lower estrogen activity via harmless nutritional means—and to do it now, while you're well—than to be forced to do it (by drastic means) by the appearance of cancer. As one cancer authority remarks: "It is well known that about one-third of breast cancer in premenopausal women is probably estrogen-dependent, since oophorectomy [removal of the ovaries] is successful in this fraction of patients."

Nature planned well in assigning the liver the task of keeping estrogen under control. This organ has unique access to both the internally produced female hormones and those that enter the body through food and medication. (There is estrogen in many foods, and estrogenic activity in drugs, in a pesticide, and even in a vitamin factor.)

As estrogen is processed by the liver, it is broken down into a series of related compounds. Each successive product exhibits less female hormone activity and, thereby, less carcinogenic (cancer-producing) effect. The final product is a hormone called estriol.

Remember that *declining female-hormone activity in any compound is correlated with reduced stimulatory action in cancer*. In pregnancy and after menopause, production of estriol rises and the occurrence of breast cancer becomes less frequent.

In certain countries—Japan, for instance— where the women tend to excrete more estriol and less estrogen, breast cancer is much more infrequent than it is in American women. But when Japanese women migrate to Hawaii, as thousands of them have, they become as susceptible as American women to the ravages of breast cancer after about a decade.

What has changed? The air they breathe, the

water they drink? Obviously, the most drastic changes occur in their diets. In their native lands, Chinese and Japanese women do not consume the staggering amount of sugar that American women, often unknowingly, ingest. Nor do they consume overprocessed breakfast cereals and fiberless white bread. Studies have not yet been made of the changes in the excretion of estriol in Japanese women who relocate to Hawaii, but I have suggested such research to the Harvard University group that has been searching for the reasons westernized Oriental women are more susceptible to cancer of the breast. My own research strongly indicates that the operative factor is the American diet.

A Lesson from Men

Oddly enough, some of our basic knowledge about the liver's effect on estrogen derives from observations of the reactions of male prisoners of war on starvation diets. Physicians confined with these men observed a definite shift toward the feminine characteristics that had developed in male heart-attack victims who had been heavily dosed with estrogen in a futile attempt to ward off subsequent attacks. (Estrogen was given in the belief that the high resistance of premenopausal women to heart disease is based solely on their high output of estrogen.)

The prisoners of war developed softer facial

hair, and thus did not need to shave as often as they previously had; and experienced loss of libido and enlargement of the breasts. When they were liberated and treated for malnourishment, these symptoms disappeared. What had happened was clear: Famine had impaired the ability of the liver to break down the female hormone. (Estrogen is manufactured in the male body, but it is present in smaller quantities than in women.) The starved soldiers were the victims of abnormally high levels of estrogen in their bodies. These levels dropped when good diet restored the ability of their livers to inactivate estrogen.

A Healthier Diet

The *Journal of the International Academy of Metabology* reported in March, 1975 on a vital experiment. Women suffering from marked premenstrual tension—water retention, severe cramps, backaches, pains in the thighs, dizziness, anxiety, and depression—were treated solely with improvements in their diets. This proved to be no panacea—*but a majority of the subjects responded with marked lessening or complete disappearance of many of the symptoms.* In addition, there was a lessening of susceptibility to cysts of the breasts and persistent cystic mastitis. Since the latter is regarded by some gynecologists as potentially precancerous,

this response may be a token of heightened
resistance to breast cancer.

The chemistry of nutrition involved, and the
dietary changes invoked to further it, were simple. In essence, the women were placed on a
high-fiber diet and the BAMBY plan. What happened is concisely stated in the abstract of the
paper in which I reported this research.

Augmented intake of vitamin B complex
and protein was used to encourage hepatic
degradation of estrogen in a group of premenopausal females, yielding significant
improvement in premenstrual tension,
dysmenorrhea, metrorrhagia, cutaneous
vascular spiders, palmar erythema, cystic
mastitis, and, in several cases, uterine
fibroid tumors. Both dietary sources and
supplements of vitamin B complex were
employed; such supplements provided significant potencies of lipotropic factors, plus
a natural source of the unknown factors of
the vitamin B complex usually derived from
desiccated liver. Protein intake was usually
derived from foods, but protein supplements were frequently employed.

Patients exhibiting the classical stigmata
of nutritional deficiencies were excluded
from the study. The results indicate that
hepatic degradation of estrogen, producing
a more favorable ratio of urinary estrogen

to estriol, may be rendered more efficient with nutritional therapies, even when applied to patients who would ordinarily be regarded as well-nourished.

One sentence in that abstract is of great significance: *"Patients exhibiting the classical stigmata of nutritional deficiencies were excluded from the study."* In other words, we chose to improve the diets of women whose diets, by all conventional standards, *needed* no improvement. Yet these same women clearly showed that their livers were controlling estrogen activity much more effectively after the changes in diet were made.

When you consider the description of the simple dietary changes that yielded so many benefits, you will realize why this chapter is part of a book on the high-fiber diet. If you follow the high-fiber diet plan, you will be increasing more than your intake of fiber. You will also be the beneficiary of a low-sugar regime, increased amounts of vitamin B complex, and more satisfactory protein intake. You will be employing *every* nutritional device to improve liver function.

We have established that the high-fiber diet helps the liver dispose of bile salts and cholesterol. At the same time, the high-fiber diet helps the liver in its control of estrogen levels. With the help of fiber you can wrap yourself in a kind of nutritional armor against the danger of undesirably high estrogen activity.

I urge you to give thought to this. If I am right about the high-fiber diet and estrogen, you will gain enormous dividends. If I am wrong, you will still earn the many other dividends improven nutrition and the high-fiber diet can give you.

A Physician's View

It is appropriate here to quote a statement made by a doctor who was in the professional group that heard and discussed a paper I wrote on nutritional management of estrogen-dependent disorders. "We already know," she said, "that the Pill causes deficiencies of five B vitamins and also causes local tissue deficiencies at the cervix. If such deficiencies impede the ability of the body to control estrogenic activity, we physicians will be remiss if we do not prescribe vitamin B complex and an excellent, high-protein diet for premenopausal patients for whom we recommend estrogen medication or contraceptives containing the hormone."

In response to this statement, I pointed out that the dietary prescription is also imperative for those women whose premenstrual tension, dysmenorrhea (painful menstruation), and cystic mastitis indicate that they are internally overdosing themselves with the hormone.

This book has revealed that many disorders of the digestive tract—from diverticular disease to bowel cancer—may be the price we pay for eating unnatural foods. What you have just read indicates that poor nutrition may also be the cause of disorders women have long considered to be the price they must pay for their biological birthright—the ability to bring children into the world.

Readers who are interested in further investigation of the relationships between diet, estrogen activity, menstrual disturbances, and estrogen-dependent cancer may wish to read the following:

Biskind, Morton. 1946. "Nutritional Therapy of Endocrine Disturbances." In *Vitamins and Hormones*. New York: Academic Press.

Black, N.M., and Leis, H.P., Jr. December 18, 1972. "Medical News." *Journal of the American Medical Association*, pp. 1483 and 1492.

Cole, Phillip. "Report to the American Cancer Society's Fourteenth Annual Science Writers' Seminar." Published by the American Cancer Society.

Fredericks, C., and Goodman, H. 1968. *Low Blood Sugar and You*. New York: Grosset and Dunlap.

Grand, Roald N. 1969. "Interview with Dr. Roy Hertz at the National Institutes of Health." Published by the American Cancer Society.

Journal of the American Medical Association. January 21, 1974, pp. 318-19.

Kast, Ludwig. "Recent Advances in Cancer Research" (lecture). Published by the New York Academy of Medicine.

Lemon, H.M., et al. June 27, 1966. "Reduced Estriol Excretion in Patients with Breast Cancer Prior to Endocrine Therapy." *Journal of the American Medical Association,* pp. 112-19.

Mecklenburg, R.S., and Lipsett, M.B. October 18, 1973. "Disappearance of Metastatic Breast Cancer After Oophorectomy." *New England Journal of Medicine,* pp. 845-46.

Sadoff, Leonard. October 18, 1973. "Letter." *New England Journal of Medicine,* pp. 863-64.

Soskin, Samuel, and Levine, Rachmiel. 1952. *Carbohydrate Metabolism.* Chicago: University of Chicago Press, p. 279.

Taylor, S.G., III. 1962. "Endocrine Ablation in Disseminated Mammary Carcinoma." *Surgical Gynecology and Obstetrics,* pp. 443-48.

Ward, H.W.C. 1973. *British Medical Journal,* no. 1, pp. 13-14.

Wotiz, Herbert H. "Report to the American Cancer Society's Fourteenth Annual Science Writers' Seminar." Published by the American Cancer Society.

18. The Constructive High-Fiber Reducing Diet

Wonder reducing diets are legion—the wonder being that you survive them! They promise to melt away a pound a day. I tell you flatly that they're dangerous. I could name half a dozen famous stars of the stage and screen who lost a hundred or more pounds in three, four, or five months—and who aren't around anymore. Their death certificates said nothing about excessively fast weight loss. They listed pneumonia, or complications after surgery, or some other ostensible illness as the cause of death, instead of the underlying and lethal factor— abrupt, severe malnutrition. But if you stil' want to lose thirty or forty pounds in a hurry, side effects be damned, you can skip this *constructive high-fiber reducing diet.*

The constructive high-fiber reducing diet has a thirty-year history of success. With it, overweight people have lost a hundred pounds and more—safely and sanely, without starvation. It carries a hidden dividend· It doesn't create the yo-yo dieter who loses a thousand pounds in twenty years—fifty pounds off and fifty pounds on each year. The yo-yo is a product of the blitz diets, for no reducing regime will create permanent weight loss if it doesn't retrain your eating habits. This the constructive high-fiber diet does. Without re-education in selecting the right foods and the right portions, the reducer inevitably goes back to his original, faulty eating habits and his original haunch, paunch, bicycle-tire-about-the-midriff, and jowl.

Constructive reduction creates no deficiency —except in calories. The constructive high-fiber reducing diet is balanced in protein values, and it contains enough fats and carbohydrates to keep body function unimpaired. By the code system it employs and the lists of permitted foods it supplies, the need for set menus and for calorie-counting is eliminated. With this diet, every effort has been made to keep vitamin-and-mineral intake at high levels. However, any diet below 2,400 calories is likely to be deficient in vitamins and minerals—that's why risk is always involved in reducing the gross intake of food. And as the calorie value of a diet drops below 1,600, it becomes increasingly difficult to maintain vitamin-and-mineral adequacy. For this reason, it is recommended that the constructive high-fiber reducing diet be supplemented with multiple vitamins, multiple minerals, and a source of the entire vitamin B complex.

Such supplements are available in pill, capsule, and liquid form from many reputable manufacturers. If taken with an additional supplement of lecithin—available in liquid, granule, and capsule form—these supplements may also help you avoid excessive loss of subcutaneous fat on the face. (Such loss makes some reducers look so cadaverous that they become discouraged and quit dieting before they've reached ideal weight.)

The assumptions behind the constructive high-fiber diet are that you, like most Americans, (a) frequently eat meals in restaurants,* (b) do little home baking, and (c) will not, therefore, be able to comply with a reducing diet that calls for bread baked with added bran, high-bran muffins, or similar special foods. For that reason, the bran added to this diet is specified in tablet form.

Bran tablets are widely available in health-food stores, usually in half-gram sizes, and two of them are roughly equivalent to a teaspoon of bran. *The recommended intake is one to two teaspoons of bran three times a day*—that is, two to four bran tablets with each meal. For those who breakfast at home, unprocessed miller's bran can be added to cereal or juice, but this kind of bran isn't very portable. The diet

---

* To make it easier to follow the constructive high-fiber diet in restaurants, sizes of portions, rather than weights, are supplied. Note that there is no calorie-counting necessary.

offers you the option of using tablets or bran in other forms.

What dividends should a reducer expect from the bran in the high-fiber reducing diet? Extravagant claims are made in some of the books on the subject—bran may decrease absorption of the foods you consume, bran may increase excretion of fat in the bowel movement, etc. I prefer to suggest that the bran simply offers the dividends in well-being discussed in the preceding chapters, including healthful changes in the bacterial flora, in stool-transit time, and in elimination. Reducing is at best a stress, not a joy; heightened well-being is a great dividend when you're losing weight. Of particular interest is the sense of fullness that comes with the bran supplement. For many reducers this is an invaluable aid—not to *will* power, but to *won't* power.

In the following menus for the constructive high-fiber reducing diet, please select foods from the appropriate lists. All lists follow the menus. Note that miller's bran may be added to juice at breakfast and powdered bran may be added to yogurt or other foods if you prefer not to use bran tablets.

FOR BREAKFAST YOU MAY EAT:

One serving of fruit or juice
One egg or egg substitute

One serving of plain yogurt

One cup of decaffeinated coffee or weak tea; no sugar, but a little milk may be added

Two to four 500-mg. (half-gram) tablets of bran with a glass of water

FOR LUNCH YOU MAY EAT:

One helping of lean meat, fish, fowl, or meat substitute

One vegetable from vegetable list "A"

One salad (from salad list)

One serving of fruit or dessert

One glass of skimmed milk or buttermilk or one cup of plain yogurt

One cup of coffee or tea (optional); no sugar, cream, or milk

Two to four 500-mg. (half-gram) tablets of bran with a glass of water

FOR DINNER YOU MAY EAT:

One cup of soup (optional)

One helping of lean meat, fish, fowl, or meat substitutes

Two vegetables from vegetable list "A" and one from vegetable list "B"

or

One vegetable from vegetable list "A" and one from vegetable list "B"

One helping of salad (from salad list)
One portion of fruit or dessert
Coffee or tea; no sugar, cream, or milk
Two to four 500-mg. (half-gram) tablets of
    bran with a glass of water

CHOOSE FOODS FROM THE LISTS
THAT FOLLOW:

DESSERTS

Fruit cocktail (with fruits from fruit list);
    small portion
Cantaloupe cocktail
Orangeade (with one and a half oranges,
    half a lemon, an egg white, and saccha-
    rine for sweetening—don't strain juice)
Milk and artificially sweetened ginger ale
    (half and half)
Milk and strawberry "soda" (half a glass
    of milk and a few large strawberries
    whipped in the blender)

EGGS AND EGG SUBSTITUTES

Plain omelet
Poached egg
Soft-boiled egg
Hard-boiled egg
Raw egg
Cottage cheese (four tablespoonfuls)
Lamb chop (one small, lean)

Lamb kidney (one)
Calves' liver (two ounces)
Mutton chop (one small, lean)
Buttermilk (one glass)
Skimmed milk (one glass)

FISH

Sea bass (1/4 pound)
Bluefish (1/4 pound)
Cod, fresh or salt (1/4 pound to 1/2 pound)
Flounder (1/4 pound to 1/2 pound)
Haddock (1/4 pound to 1/2 pound)
Halibut (1/4 pound)
Kingfish (1/4 pound)
Pike (1/4 pound)
Porgy (1/4 pound)
Red snapper (1/4 pound)
Scallops (2/3 cup, raw measurement)
Shrimp (2/3 cup)
Smelt (1/4 pound)
Weakfish (1/4 pound)
Clams, round (ten to twelve)
Crab meat (one crab or 3/4 cup flakes)
Lobster (1/2 small lobster or one cup flakes)
Mussels (four large or eight small)
Oysters (twelve large)

Note: Portions of fish are more generous than meat portions, and fish is frequently less costly in today's market. Fish protein is nutritional equivalent of meat and fowl.

FRUITS

Orange (small)
Grapefruit (half, medium size)
Apple (small)
Pineapple (two average slices)
Peach (one)
Cantaloupe (half, medium size)
Melons (two-inch section of average size melon)
Tangerine (large)
Berries (½ cup)
Apricots (two, medium size)
Grapes (twelve)
Cherries (ten)
Pear (medium size)
Plums (two)
Nectarines (three)
Persimmon (half, small)
Fruit juices:
grapefruit, orange (unsweetened; six ounces)

MEATS

Lean beefsteak (¼ pound about one inch thick, 2½ inches square)
Roast beef (two slices, about three inches square, ¼ inch thick)

Beef liver (one slice, three inches square, ½ inch thick)

Beef tongue (two average slices)

Beef kidney (¼ pound)

Hamburger (¼ pound)

Calves' liver (¼ pound)

Lamb kidneys (two, average size)

Lamb chop (one, about two inches square, ½ inch thick)

Roast lamb (one slice, 3½ inches square, ¼ inch thick)

Mutton chops (two, medium size)

Boiled mutton (one slice, four inches square, ½ inch thick)

Roast veal (one slice, three inches by two inches, ¼ inch thick)

Veal cutlet (one, average size)

Veal kidneys (two, average size)

Chicken, white meat (two slices, four inches square, cut very thin)

Chicken, broiler (½ medium size)

Chicken gizzards (two, average size)

Chicken livers (two, medium size)

MEAT SUBSTITUTES

Cottage cheese (2/3 cup)

Eggs—poached or omelet (two eggs)

Buttermilk (two cups)

Whole milk (one cup)

Skimmed milk (two cups)

SALADS

Tossed greens
Watercress and lettuce
Radish and watercress
Celery and cabbage
Pimento and greens
Baked stuffed tomato (with cottage cheese
    and chopped celery)

One teaspoonful of salad dressing may be
used. Divide between lunch and dinner, if
salads are eaten twice daily; use vinegar or
lemon juice to augment.

SOUPS

Consomme
Clear vegetable soup
Beef broth
Chicken or mutton broth
Other clear soups

Note: No creamed soups or soups containing milk, vegetables, meat, or cereals are
allowed.

VEGETABLE LIST "A"

Asparagus (fresh or canned; eight)
String beans (½ cup)
Wax beans (½ cup)
Beet greens (two heaping tablespoons)

Broccoli (one five-inch stalk)
Brussels sprouts (½ cup)
Cabbage, cooked (½ cup)
Cabbage, raw (¾ cup, shredded)
Cauliflower (½ cup)
Celery (five stalks)
Chard (½ cup)
Chicory (½ cup)
Eggplant (½ cup)
Endive (ten medium stalks)
Green pepper (one, medium size)
Kohlrabi (two heaping tablespoonfuls)
Leeks, chopped (one-third cup)
Lettuce (ten leaves)
Radishes (five, medium size)
Sauerkraut (½ cup)
Spinach (½ cup)
Tomatoes, fresh (one)
Tomatoes, canned (½ cup)
Tomato juice (½ cup)
Watercress (ten pieces)

VEGETABLE LIST "B"

Beets (two heaping tablespoons)
Carrots (two heaping tablespoons)
Chives (six)
Dandelion greens (three heaping table-
spoons)
Kale (two heaping tablespoons)
Onion (one, small size)

Parsnips (two heaping tablespoons)
Peas (two heaping tablespoons)
Pumpkin (three heaping tablespoons)
Rutabaga (two heaping tablespoons)
Squash (two heaping tablespoons)
Turnips (two heaping tablespoons)

Special Notes

Artificial sweeteners—If you are concerned with ominous reports on sugar substitutes but can't dispense with them until the conflicting findings are reconciled, it is best to stop the use of these artificial sweeteners completely every third week; this permits the body to clear the residues from its systems.

Water consumption—Bran is thirsty; in fact, this is one of the bases for its normalizing effect on elimination. Do drink a glass of water at any meal where bran is used. This means three glasses per day in this plan, and more may be used, if that is your habit, but *not less*. Don't be deterred by the numerous adverse reports on the quality of the drinking water in many large American cities. Simply find room in your budget for the purchase of pure spring mineral water. There are a number of brands of mineral water on the market; they originate from some of America's most famous spas.

Extra allowance of margarine—Unsaturated fat, like that supplied by most margarines, helps the body to metabolize the hard, stored fat that is sometimes impervious to weight loss. A level teaspoonful of margarine may be used at lunch or dinner on your vegetables—or, if you prefer, you may replace the margarine with an extra teaspoonful of salad oil on your salad at lunch or dinner. Note that the oils in health-food stores tend to be free of undesirable additives that other oils may contain.

Supplements—Take your bran at the beginning of the meal to give it time to help you to feel sated. Remember that the amount of supplementary bran needed differs from person to person—some people may require less than I suggest; some may require more. The criteria by which you judge are simple. If the amount of bran is right, elimination will become easy and the stool will become progressively more and more odor-free. This effect will be accelerated if the suggestions concerning the use of yogurt are followed. If for any reason yogurt is unavailable, you can purchase tablets of the lactobacillus organism in concentrated form.

Vitamin, mineral, and B complex supplements should be taken with food, not on an empty stomach, and they should be taken at breakfast or lunch. For many people, these supplements provide a lift in energy that is wonderful during the day but they may interfere with sleep if they are used at night.

While most people are familiar with multiple vitamin-and-mineral supplements, few are acquainted with *chelated* mineral supplements, and still fewer know how to use a *natural* B-complex supplement properly. Chelated multiple mineral supplements present the minerals in a form that the body can utilize more efficiently. Natural vitamin B complex can be obtained from brewer's yeast or desiccated liver. The dose? This is food, not medicine, so "a handful" is probably the most appropriate answer! A dose of half a dozen or a dozen tablets is probably good for most people. The point is that there are unknown vitamins that we haven't learned to synthesize. They come to you only from a natural source, and brewer's yeast and liver are such sources. (Note: If you're an allergic person, these supplements should be used only once every fourth or fifth day, to minimize the possibility of your being sensitized to one of their many natural nutrients.)

That lecithin supplements will help you avoid that "pinched look" that comes with the loss of subcutaneous fat in your face is *not* based on mere theory. Dr. Harry Swartz and I, in controlled research some twenty years ago, demonstrated this effect in several hundred reducers.

Lecithin is most conveniently used in nineteen-grain capsules; take two after each meal. Some reducers prefer the granules, but these are difficult to use when the diet doesn't include cereal or another convenient vehicle for this form of lecithin. Others get their lecithin in an oil base and take it by the spoonful. Lecithin, incidentally, isn't a drug. It's a food factor, natural to the body—in fact, manufactured by the liver—and it has potent effects on fats and fat metabolism.

A final word on supplements: Don't let the long list discourage you. For most people the rewards match the effort, and the prevention of deficiency is important. If you're not an enthusiastic user of pills and such, confine yourself to the multiple vitamin, multiple mineral, and bran concentrates. Dividends will still accrue, and your constructive high-fiber reducing diet will still be effective if you're in normal health. This qualifying phrase *doesn't* mean that food supplements, lecithin, and bran are dangerous for the ill. It simply means that self-treatment is accurately described as having an unqualified physician taking care of you.

Naturally, the constructive high-fiber diet is aimed at people of normal health who are moderately overweight. If you have health problems, the diet should be followed and the supplements of bran, vitamins, minerals, and B complex used *under your physician's direction.*

How to Stay Slim

When your diet has brought you to normal weight, increase your milk intake to two full glasses a day, and use as many of the leafy vegetables in vegetable list "A" as you wish. If you don't gain—or you continue to lose—you can then increase your intake of whole-grain bread. (Useful tip: Brown-rice crackers are available in the supermarket. It takes ten of them to equal one slice of bread, and this certainly gives you an illusion of unlimited, even riotous, eating. And they *are* whole grain, meaning that they provide natural fiber—it's rice bran.) If you still don't gain, the root and starchy vegetables may now be added—gently, please—and, with them, a little more butter or margarine or salad oil. The supplements to the diet—the vitamins, minerals, B complex, bran, and lecithin—should be continued.

I hope to see less of you.

19. The Combination High-Fiber, Low-Carbohydrate Reducing Diet

In Chapter 12 I described adverse reactions to the high intake of sugar, and emphasized individual differences in sugar tolerances. We are about to find that those who wish to lose weight have the same differences in tolerances for *all* carbohydrates.

There are three schools of thought about sugar and starch in the American diet. First we have the establishment view, voiced by professors of nutrition obligated for grants and donations to the very industries that process starch and sugar or use highly milled carbohydrates in their own products. One professor of nutrition at a great university (which has been the recipient of millions of dollars in gifts from manufacturers of processed cereals, flour, and sugar) will state in press interviews that he sees nothing wrong in taking 20 per cent of your calories from sugar alone. He will indicate that getting even 25 per cent of your calories from this foodless food would be fine!

Vehemently opposed to that philosophy are the physicians, nutritionists, and biochemists who are aware that such a high intake of sugar (or of processed starch) may contribute to gout, strokes, circulatory disorders, heart disease, constipation, varicosities, appendicitis, diverticular disease, and other disorders of sugar-saturated modern man.

Within this group, though, you will find such imperfect unanimity that there might as well be two groups. In the forefront of one are medical men like Dr. John Yudkin, who believes that man has never wholly adapted to high-sugar, high-starch foods, and should return to his original hunter-herdsman diet—high in fats and proteins, very low in carbohydrates. The opposing school—represented by Dr. Thomas L. Cleave—agrees that man has not adapted to concentrated, highly processed carbohydrates, which come to him in an unnatural form. But to the medical men and nutritionists of Cleave's school of thought, the problem is overindulgence.

Many years ago, I studied these opposing philosophies and made a decision. I based it on clinical observation of the responses of *people*, both sick and well, to various types of therapeutic and maintenance diets. I do not present this decision to you in the belief that I'm always right. (It's just that those who disagree with me are always wrong!) I do believe, however, that logic is strongly on my side.

Everyone in nutrition who is objective will recognize that overprocessing of carbohydrates —resulting in the loss of nutrients, bran, and the germ of whole grains—is biologically insane. Those of us who are sensitive to individual differences in nutritional needs and tolerances know that there are those who tolerate reasonable amounts of starches and sugars, and those who simply don't. Objective nutritionists are also aware that overprocessed carbohydrates, unless consumed in miniscule amounts, are a stress on the human organism.

I am saying, in short, that I don't subscribe to the belief that no one's body has adapted to the high level of sugars and starches in our modern diet. The evidence suggests strongly that some people have adapted—but some obviously haven't, and won't. You yourself may have unconsciously recognized such differences. You frequently hear the remark, "When I even *smell* a cake baking, I gain weight. Other people can gorge on fattening foods and nothing happens." And you've undoubtedly heard of—or known— the family in which, *on the same intake of carbohydrates,* one member has rampant tooth decay and another seems to have total dental immunity. Not only does tooth enamel differ, but so does resistance to cavities induced by carbohydrates.

Conventional Weight-Loss Plans

But a virtually unrecognized tolerance difference appears in overweight people's reactions to carbohydrates. There is a substantial group that can't reduce on conventional low-calorie weight-loss diets because such diets—like American diets generally—consist of 50 per cent carbohydrates. These people do well on a diet supplying much less starch and sugar, even when their total calorie intake is higher than it is on a conventional weight-loss diet. And this is the group that so upsets the orthodox doctor or nutritionist.

Placed on a conventional 1,200-calorie diet, these people either don't lose weight—or manage somehow, in violation of all the laws of calorie-input versus calorie-expenditure, to gain weight. Placed on a 1,400- or 1,600-calorie diet with starches and sugars cut down much more than they are in the usual reducing diet, they are successful in losing weight—despite the generous portions of protein and fat allowed. It isn't the number of calories that poses the problem to these people—it is the fact that 50 per cent of their calories had come from starch and sugar, however much the gross intake might be trimmed to fit within a 1,000- or 1,200-calorie regime.

The non-adapters to the conventional weight-reducing diet have well-defined, unique biochemical characteristics; they are different from the rest of the overweight population. They are excessively efficient in converting starch and sugar into stored fat, which is then retained by the body in a form that is reluctant to yield to ordinary weight-loss techniques.

Some people tend to retain salt in direct relationship to the amount of carbohydrate they eat. Storing salt creates the tendency to store water and, since reducing is a process of turning body fat into water (among other things), it's obvious that people who retain water will retain *excess weight* in the form of water. Therefore, they will not slim down on a conventional reducing diet with its usual high amount of daily carbohydrate intake.

The conventional medical approach to this problem is symptomatic treatment, usually with diuretics—drugs that force the body to expel fluid. This approach gives only temporary help, for the problem of water storage will continue until carbohydrate intake is reduced to the level of the person's tolerance for it.

The Low-Carbohydrate Diet

Those of us experienced with *low-carbohydrate diets* use five devices to help reducers:

1. We recommend the diet for healthy, if

overweight, people whose physicians have not recommended low-cholesterol diets.

2. We divide daily menus into six meals. The body is less efficient in utilizing small meals. This helps weight loss and improves the efficiency of the body's management of both cholesterol and glucose.

3. We give about 20 per cent of the total fat intake in the form of polyunsaturated fats or oils. These tend to lower, rather than raise, blood cholesterol. Such vegetable fats also induce some of the stored, hard fat in the body to participate in the chain of metabolic processes that ultimately burns it into water and carbon dioxide. This type of food simultaneously lessens the tendency to salt retention, so that excessive amounts of the water resulting from oxidation of fat are not stored in the tissues. (This is a way of saying that the low-carbohydrate diet has a natural diuretic effect.) The mitigation of salt retention yields another dividend. There is no need to forbid the *moderate* use of salt or, for that matter, any other type of seasoning.*

* This license is revoked for those with hypertension or a tendency toward it and for those whose physicians have placed them on low-salt diets. In such cases, all other seasonings can be used—subject to your doctor's wishes—save celery salt, garlic salt, monosodium glutamate, and any other spices in which salt is an ingredient.

I should explain here that the phrase "low carbohydrate" does not mean dropping to zero or ten or twenty grams of starches daily. I approximate sixty grams in the menus that follow. (The conventional weight-reducing diet allows for about one hundred fifty grams of carbohydrates.) We're aware that there are those who function well and reduce very rapidly on less carbohydrate and those who feel well and lose weight rapidly on more. However, at sixty grams daily, the carbohydrate intake is low enough to let the majority lose weight, and high enough that the unpleasant side effects of zero carbohydrate diets are averted. For the technically minded, the preceding remark means that given a choice between slower reduction or greater degree of ketosis, I have otped for conservative rates of weight loss.

4. The diet is supplemented with vitamins that not only help protect against deficiency but also aid in fat utilization. For this purpose, we use a vitamin-B-complex concentrate that is high in choline and inositol. Added effectiveness can be achieved by the use of a lecithin supplement. If vitamin E concentrates are added, one of the effects (previously mentioned) may be more selectiveness in the reducing process—retention of subcutaneous fat on the face so you avoid that cadaverous look, and

less retention of the stubborn bulges that often resist weight loss.

5. Ordinarily, since bran and fiber are components of foods rich in carbohydrate, a high-fiber, low-carbohydrate diet would seem to be a contradiction in terms. It's made possible by three devices. First, all the recommended carbohydrates are of the unprocessed types, which are bran sources. Second, emphasis is placed on consumption of salads and whole fruits and vegetables, which are *not* high in carbohydrates but *do* supply fiber. Third, we employ a bran supplement, either miller's bran added to recipes or bran tablets. Bran is a modest source of carbohydrate—it contains about six grams per tablespoonful—so that even those who need the maximum amount of bran will not be breaking through the carbohydrate ceiling if they continue to use a lot of bran.

Astonishing Success

In the first two weeks on this diet, your weight loss may be dramatic. I have observed losses of as much as fourteen pounds in that period. A large percentage of that may be water—the diet itself is naturally diuretic because it persuades your body not to retain salt. After the first two weeks, not only will the weight loss slow to a reasonable figure, but you may strike plateaus where nothing seems to be happening. If you persist, however, weight loss will usually resume.

It goes without saying that the diet isn't successful for 100 per cent of those who follow it. Nutritional science is as devoid of panaceas as any other discipline. In the main, though, the low-carbohydrate regime has an astonishing record of success, considering that those who try it are frequently those for whom the orthodox, calorie-restricted diet has failed.

Two points must be re-emphasized. First, without the stipulated amount of unsaturated fat in the diet, it is likely that nothing will happen. Secondly, if you don't divide the day's food intake into six small rather than three large meals, reduction will be achieved only at a pedestrian pace. This, naturally, could be demoralizing.

A final note before you take the plunge: Don't be put off by the surprising amount of food permitted in these menus. That's one of the dividends of a low-carbohydrate diet. Herman Taller was right when he said calories don't count; he meant that *sources* of calories were more important than the arithmetic. The years have verified his findings.

The medical pioneer of the nineteenth century, William Harvey, is believed to have prescribed a low-carbohydrate diet, for one of Har-

vey's grossly overweight patients published a
diary in which he triumphantly recorded that, for
the first time in his life, he was able to lose
weight. The Earl of Salisbury, in the 1890s, suc-
cessfully used the low-carbohydrate diet. You
commemorate that triumph when you call a
hamburger a "Salisbury steak," which was a part
of the nobleman's high-protein, low-carbohydrate
menus. The diet was also used by Pennington at
the Dupont Clinic, where he pronounced it a
successful method of weight loss. Gordon, of
the University of Wisconsin Medical School,
found the diet highly successful, and recorded
his observations in a paper in the *Journal* of the
American Medical Association—which never
stopped the A.M.A. from denouncing the concept as invalid.

Some Dos and Don'ts

In the menus for the combination high-fiber
low-carbohydrate reducing diet, there are no ab-
solutes in choice of foods, provided that you
exchange like for like—carbohydrate for carbohydrate, protein for protein, unsaturated fat for
unsaturated fat, saturated fat for saturated fat.
This means you may interchange eggs for
meat, meat for fish, fowl for cheese, etc.; you
may choose brown-rice crackers in the stipulated amount for the whole-wheat bread or

whole-rye or whole-corn bread. You may choose vegetable (salad) oil in place of margarine. But *don't* take more bread in exchange for less meat. *Don't* substitute butter or lard for vegetable oil, and *don't* skimp on fish to "make room" for a forbidden dessert. If you do, you'll defeat your diet and stop your weight loss.

In exchanging one food for another of the same type, there *is* one thing you should be careful of. If you don't like or don't tolerate milk, yogurt, or cheese, and choose to substitute other proteins for these—meat, fish, or fowl, for example—you will create a deficit in calcium, which is provided by the dairy foods but is poorly supplied by other proteins. If you choose not to use dairy products, a calcium supplement—bone meal, dolomite, or calcium orotate (the most effective)—is a wise protection.

The use of salad oil and margarine in the low-carbohydrate menus is *not* optional. You may consider it strange that you are required to use about five teaspoonfuls of such high-calorie fats daily, but please remember that this diet has nothing to do with calories. Unsaturated fat is needed to make the diet effective, to help not only with weight loss but also with losing the bulges that ordinarily evade the effect of weight loss.

Use about five teaspoonfuls of vegetable fats daily. This doesn't mean hydrogenated fats, even if they are of vegetable origin. It means mayonnaise, salad oil—preferably uncooked—and margarine. It's preferable to use at least three teaspoonfuls of oil on your daily salads and derive the other two teaspoonfuls from the other fats listed. Wheat-germ oil is fine, if you prefer it. Any other vegetable oil (*except olive oil*) is approved, so long as it doesn't contain BHA or BHT.

Avoid all forms of sugar—soft drinks, sugar-sweetened juices, sugar-packed or syrup-packed canned and frozen foods. Avoid also honey, molasses, and other foods rich in carbohydrates, such as cookies, pretzels, crackers, potato chips, cakes, and popcorn. Use salt substitutes as you wish or as your physician instructs. Use sugar substitutes within reason. You may have unsweetened whole gelatin, incorporating permitted fruits in permitted amounts, as a dessert. Vinegar, spices, herbs, and lemon juice are allowed.

Take your supplements—vitamin B complex, vitamin E, lecithin, bran. If your dietary history is shaky, add a multiple vitamin-and-mineral supplement.

If you're a compulsive late-night refrigerator raider, use a small glass of a dry wine an hour before dinner and an hour before bedtime. But don't use it if you don't really need it.

Other rules are minor, but logical and important. Stay within the limits of carbohydrate allowed. Interchange leafy vegetables as you choose, but don't substitute potatoes—high in starch—for spinach, which is low in starch. Fruits are relatively rich in sugar, and portions of these *must* be held to the limits set in the menus. But generally fruits are interchangeable, too, as long as they're listed as permissible.

If you don't want to add bran to recipes where it's specified, your other option is the use of bran tablets, as described in Chapter 13. This is a must, not only because of the benefits of bran that you have come to appreciate in reading this book, but because a reducing diet obviously minimizes the amount of food residue, and may thereby induce constipation.

You will recall that you should begin with a teaspoonful of bran daily and work your way up. Some people do well on three teaspoonfuls, in divided dose, daily; some need twice as much; and some may have to graduate to three tablespoonfuls daily. It has already been estimated for you that a half-gram bran tablet is equivalent to a half teaspoonful of bran. (Two to a teaspoonful, six to a tablespoonful is the rough scale of equivalents.) There will be a difference in the volume (and weight) of finely ground and coarsely ground brans, and the latter is more effective for some people. The criteria by which you judge which bran is best for you have been described in Chapter 13.

TYPICAL LOW-CARBOHYDRATE
MEALS AND SNACKS

BREAKFAST

Grapefruit half

Poached egg with two pork or beef sausages (no BHA or BHT)

Half slice of whole-wheat, whole-rye, or whole-corn bread with 1 level teaspoonful of highly unsaturated margarine (commercial rye bread is like white bread—seek whole-grain rye)

Beverage of choice—coffee or decaffeinated coffee, herb or regular tea; use cream and artificial sweetener, if desired

MORNING BOOSTER

Skim milk (one cup)

Creamed cottage cheese (¼ cup) with added bran, well stirred*

LUNCH

Clear soup (optional)

Chicken salad (with approximately four ounces of chicken and one or two teaspoons mayonnaise, on lettuce, chicory or escarole—unlimited amounts—plus chopped celery, and sliced tomatoes)

---

* If bran tablets are not being used, or if you need more bran than is supplied by the tablets.

Green or wax beans or other vegetable from
   approved list
Brown-rice crackers (five) with ½ teaspoon
   margarine, **or** brown-rice cake (obtainable in health-food stores)
Beverage of choice

AFTERNOON SNACK

Yogurt (½ cup) with added bran, well
   stirred*
Your favorite cheese (one ounce)—**not**
   "cheese food"—with one small whole-
   wheat cracker

DINNER

Clear soup (optional)
Tomato juice (four ounces)
Steak (¼ pound)
Cauliflower with one teaspoon margarine
Tossed salad, vinegar-and-oil dressing†
Strawberries and half-and-half (small
   amount) with optional artificial sweet-
   ener
Beverage of choice

EVENING SNACK

Skim milk or yogurt (½ cup) with added
   bran*

---

* If bran tablets are not being used, or if you need more
bran than is supplied by the tablets.
† No limit on salad portions.

157

Leftover chicken, cheese, meat, or fish (one ounce) **or** a small portion of peanut or other nut butter on two brown-rice crackers, one brown-rice cake, or one whole-grain cracker

Your vegetables will be selected from the following list. Eat a daily minimum of two cups, total, up to a maximum of four cups.

APPROVED VEGETABLES

Vegetables marked with a dot are good sources of vitamin C, often rich in other nutritional values, and should be emphasized if they please your palate. Of course, the vitamins in your multiple vitamin supplement will protect you even if you're determined not to eat anything that's good for you.

Asparagus	Kohlrabi
Avocado	Leeks
●Broccoli	●Kale
Brussels sprouts	●Mustard
Cabbage	●Spinach
Celery	●Turnip greens
Chicory	Lettuce
Cucumbers	Mushrooms
Escarole	Radishes
Eggplant	Sauerkraut
Green pepper	String beans

- Beet greens   Green or wax beans
- Chard   Tomatoes
- Collards   Tomato juice
- Dandelion   Summer squash
  Endive   Watercress

APPROVED FRUITS

Take two servings of *fruit* daily, in amounts listed. Those marked with a dot are good sources of vitamin C. Fresh, canned, cooked, or frozen fruits may be used, if they're free of added sugar—artificially sweetened fruit is O.K., though. Don't peel fresh fruit—peels are fiber sources.

Apple	(small)
Applesauce	(½ cup)
Apricots, fresh	(two medium)
Apricots, dried	(four halves)
Banana	(½ small)
Blackberries	(one cup)
Blueberries	(2/3 cup)
• Cantaloupe	(¼ of six-inch melon)
Cherries	(ten large)
Cranberries	(one cup)
Dates	(two)
Figs, fresh	(two large)
Figs, dried	(one small)
• Grapefruit	(½ small)
• Grapefruit juice	(½ cup)

Grapes	(twelve large)
Grape juice	(¼ cup)
Honeydew melon	(⅛ medium)
Mango	(one small)
Nectarine	(one medium)
•Orange	(one small)
•Orange juice	(½ cup)
Papaya	(1/3 medium)
Peach	(one medium)
Pear	(one small)
Persimmon	(½ small)
Pineapple	(½ cup)
Pineapple juice	(1/3 cup)
Plums	(two medium)
Prunes	(two medium)
Raspberries	(one cup)
Rhubarb	(one cup)
•Strawberries	(one cup)
Tangerine	(one cup)
Watermelon	(one cup)

All fruits and vegetables, whether served uncooked or cooked, peeled or unpeeled, should be thoroughly washed before consumption. Pesticide residues help no one and can be reduced significantly by washing.

On the Low-Carbohydrate Diet . . .

Don't use vegetable oil for frying. There is nothing wrong with fried foods if they're properly prepared, but high temperatures may change the characteristics of the polyunsaturated fats on which this diet depends. Oil may be gently heated in the preparation of such dishes as spinach wilted in hot oil, but keep the oil below the smoking point.

Protein substitutions may be made as follows. A quarter of a cup of creamed or uncreamed cottage cheese, farmer cheese, or pot cheese may be substituted for an ounce of meat. Approximately two ounces of meat, raw weight, may be replaced with an egg. An ounce of cheddar or other American-type cheese, or the equivalent in other types, can replace about two ounces of meat, raw weight. Peanut butter is a good source of protein, but it is also a good source of carbohydrate, and the commercial varieties contain saturated fat. Even if it's one of your favorite snack foods, eat no more than one tablespoonful of peanut butter weekly.

Some final words about supplements: The high-B-complex supplement should be used in the label-designated amount. Be sure each dose you take contains at least half a gram of choline and a quarter of a gram of inositol. With vitamin-and-mineral supplements, any good product will do; take yours in the label-designated dose.

Vitamin E should be used in the form of mixed tocopherols (don't take just alpha-tocopherol alone). The potency will be measured in terms of the alpha form, and should be from 100 to 200 units daily.

Lecithin is available in granules, but this will probably not be a convenient form in the absence of cereals with which to mix them. Nineteen-grain lecithin capsules are available, and the supplementary amount is one to two; take them after each meal (three to six daily). Finally, a calcium supplement should supply you with a gram of calcium daily.

When you just can't resist temptation, strawberries are probably the lowest of fruits in carbohydrate, and they are also an excellent source of vitamin C. If you must cheat, a small bowl of strawberries, or a handful tossed into the blender with your allotment of one cup of skimmed milk, should satisfy you. Tomato juice is the lowest of the staple juices in carbohydrate. Your scale will tell you rather promptly if your backsliding threatens your reducing.

There are many recipes for low-carbohydrate desserts, some of them with low-carbohydrate whipped toppings and many of them luscious. But, inevitably, they rest heavily on artificial sweeteners, consumption of which in large amounts I am not willing to encourage until the controversy concerning the safety of these sugar substitutes is firmly resolved. I do not recommend the several brands of artificially sweetened gelatin desserts either, for none of these is innocent of coal-tar food dyes and artificial flavor, and I have grown increasingly convinced that the additive you don't swallow never makes you ill.

You will find, as your experience with the low-carbohydrate diet accumulates, that tolerance for starches and sugars does in fact vary from person to person, and that you may be able to add an extra portion of fruit (with cheese, if you like—that ceiling is flexible) as dessert. Or you may be able to tolerate the extra carbohydrate in good, high-protein cookies or muffins, recipes for which will be found in cookbooks by Beatrice Trum Hunter and Adelle Davis, as well as in this book. In the interim, be patient with those of us who are not deaf to your plea for a sop to your sweet tooth, but who aren't blind, either, to the very real potential harm of chemical sweeteners used in excess.

20. For Those Determined to Remain Healthy

A great biochemist and nutritionist, Dr. Roger Williams, has said we never achieve optimal nutrition—that the best possible diet represents a compromise. Then, too, we never achieve optimal health. My copy of the Funk and Wagnalls Encyclopedia says that health is an optimal functioning of the organism, and that it is *never* achieved. These thoughts of compromise should be kept in mind as we try to bring our diet up to the level of the rural Africans' in supporting resistance to disease. We can be consoled with the realization that *any* improvement in our nutrition and *any* heightening of our immunities will be an improvement the body will gratefully receive.

Our goals seem simple enough. We want more bran in our foods; we want to restore wheat germ to the flour products that have lost it, and to add additional amounts to the foods that contain it; we want a daily intake of yogurt to speed the process of acquiring a "friendly" bacterial flora; we want to increase our intake of minerals and vitamins. Those goals are achieved by adding bran and wheat germ to our recipes, by eating (plain, unflavored) yogurt daily, and by selecting our foods more intelligently. It is feasible to take bran in tablet form, to use a multiple vitamin-and-mineral supplement, and to hasten the growth of a favorable type of bowel bacteria by the use of lactic-acid yeast.

In adding bran to your recipes, you profit by the added fiber and nutrients of this long-neglected fraction of wheat. By choosing whole-grain breads and cereals and baking with whole-grain flour, you draw upon additional fiber. In the natural sources of bran, however, there is also the natural germ, and its values are complementary to those of bran. And remember that wheat germ has unique properties that are not shared by bran, some of which have already been described for you.

There are a number of considerations that will determine what methods you will use, as an individual, to improve your diet. If you do little cooking and less baking, then bran tablets are obviously the most convenient way to raise your fiber intake. If you breakfast at home, you can add miller's bran to your (good-to-begin-with) cereals, or to berries or other fruit. Or you can add bran to cream and thick soups or stir it into plain yogurt, with or without added fruit. For a larger plus, add a teaspoonful of full-fat wheat germ to your cereal along with your bran, or use wheat germ itself as a cereal and add bran. Wheat germ is the most nutritious natural cereal available, high in values poorly supplied by many diets. Oatmeal is also an excellent cereal, and is a good vehicle for bran and wheat germ; so is Wheatena, and so is any brand of shredded wheat that does not contain BHA or BHT.

You can see your physician to obtain a supply of lactic-acid yeast—this is available to your doctor from the Standard Process Company. He can also recommend compressed tablets of the "friendly" lactobacilli.

Brewer's yeast, wheat germ, and bran are available in health-food stores, and wheat germ is also available in grocery stores. Bran purchased in a grocery store tends to be processed, heat-treated, and formed into flakes. Raw bran is nutritionally preferable, cheaper, and devoid of additives. Do remember that wheat germ is highly perishable when it's full-fat, and is best bought vacuum-packed. Refrigerate it once the bottle has been opened. Bran is more stable but it, too, should be refrigerated.

Use brewer's yeast as a supplementary source of vitamin B complex, minerals, the glucose-tolerance factor, and Factor 3, which aids in the utilization of vitamin E. Don't accept torula yeast, which is less valuable.

When you're feeding a family, remember the

Latin phrase "*De gustibus non disputandum est.*" It means there is no accounting for taste. A head-on approach in administering supplements of bran and other nutritious goodies may invite nothing but belligerent rejection. Few people—even those with long experience in cooking for families—really appreciate the emotional climate around food habits. The most famous illustration of this can be found in the story about the physician who discovered that prescribing raw liver three times daily would halt the ravages of pernicious anemia. His patients announced that they'd taken a vote, and the majority had agreed that they preferred to die rather than eat uncooked liver three times daily.

Certainly many Americans would rather perish than eat anything that threatens to benefit them. As an experienced nutritionist who for decades has struggled with entrenched food habits, I tell you that the ultimate and fatal mistake is the head-on approach. It will invite rejection, and that is why I take a dim view of books in which bran enthusiasts suggest addition of fiber to hamburgers, meatballs, spaghetti sauce, and meat loaf. With the exception of meat loaf, I can tell you—again, based on experience—that your family will detect "foreign" ingredients if you add enough of them to be nutritionally significant.

What to do? It is tempting to suggest that you add bran and wheat germ to prepared cake, pancake, and waffle mixes. I hate to appear to endorse packaged mixes, for many of them are so full of preservatives, anti-oxidants, emulsifiers, surfactants, artificial flavors, and coal-tar colors that I often salute the technologists for leaving room in the box for the normal ingredients. For most of these commercial products, there is no way to go, nutritionally speaking, but up! So, if you insist on using mixes because they are convenient, you can certainly begin by adding two teaspoonfuls of bran and one of wheat germ to each cupful of the raw mix. Increase these portions gradually, in succeeding batches. Don't go overboard. Many novitiates, once their initial timidity or cynicism is overcome, overload recipes with bran and wheat germ, and wind up with products that quite literally weigh a ton.

When you disdain mixes and start baking from scratch, you will find that you can add a teaspoonful of wheat germ and two of bran to each cup of flour in your basic recipe. As time goes on and you gain experience, you can add larger amounts. A bran muffin, obviously, can be heavily fortified. Home-baked English muffins—actually, any of the "sour" recipes—will lend themselves to high percentages of bran and wheat germ. Both whole-wheat and white breads can be so fortified. If you are a white-bread baker, I shall suggest a variation in the recipe that turns out a much more nutritious and flavorful loaf than you ordinarily encounter in cookbooks. Read on.

21. Introducing Some High-Fiber Recipes

For the family willing to lend only stinted co-operation to the whole idea of a high-fiber diet, there is a quick and easy way to add bran and wheat germ to the diet. This recipe originated in England, which explains why, to the American palate, the high-fiber result may recall the hard-tack of old sailing days. Nonetheless, this recipe could solve the problem if your family balks at changes in familiar dishes.

Bran and Wheat Germ Crackers

½ cup of miller's bran
5/8 cup gluten flour
⅛ cup stone-ground whole-wheat flour
¼ cup sesame seeds
4 heaping teaspoons full-fat wheat germ
½ cup of water
½ teaspoonful iodized salt
¼ teaspoon baking soda

Preheat oven at 350°. Mix all dry ingredients

very thoroughly, add water, and mix well until a soft dough is produced. Roll dough on a floured surface to about 1/8-inch thickness. Use a knife to cut dough into rectangles about two inches by four inches in size. Place dough on well-greased cookie sheet and bake for ten minutes. Lower oven temperature to 300°, and bake about ten minutes more, or until the crackers are crisp. Cheese, garlic, onion, or any of a number of spices (such as caraway) may be added to taste.

Yield: About twenty crackers

A little over three grams of fiber will be provided by each of these crackers. The object is to increase fiber intake to about fifteen grams daily—"about," because the amount will vary from person to person.

A more succulent recipe, high in bran and wheat germ, is for—

Raised Bran Muffins

Stir one to three packages of baker's yeast, crumbled, into one cup of yogurt that is at room temperature. Add and lightly stir:

    3 tablespoons of dark molasses
    1 egg
    3 tablespoons of bacon drippings

Now, sift in:

1 cup of bran
1 cup of whole-wheat pastry flour
½ cup of wheat germ
⅓ cup of powdered nonfat milk
1¼ teaspoonfuls of iodized salt
½ cup of nuts—your choice of variety

Stir well. Drop from tablespoon into greased muffin tins until receptacles are half filled, let rise until double in bulk, and bake at 350° for about twenty minutes.

Here is an easy and delicious biscuit recipe that combines bran with wheat germ and whole-grain flour:

Bran Biscuits

1 cup whole-wheat, unbleached, or enriched
flour
1 cup whole bran, **or** ½ cup each whole
bran and wheat germ
½ teaspoon salt
¼ cup skim-milk solids
2½ teaspoons double-acting baking powder
4 tablespoons chilled solid shortening, lard,
margarine, or bacon grease
½ cup milk

Mix all dry ingredients together. Cut in shortening with pastry blender or two knives. Add milk and stir with a fork. Dough will be soft. Pat it on waxed paper to ½-inch thickness, cut with floured biscuit cutter, and place on greased cookie sheet—or add a little more milk and drop by the spoonful onto sheet or into greased muffin tins. Bake at 425° for fifteen to eighteen minutes.

Yield: sixteen biscuits. Don't split them; eat them whole.

For families habituated to white bread, this formula, devised by my friend and mentor, Dr. Clive McKay, offers a succulent and much more nutritious loaf.

Cornell Bread Formula

For each cup of flour, place in the measuring cup one tablespoon each of soy flour and nonfat dry milk powder, plus one teaspoon of wheat germ. Fill the remainder of the cup with unbleached flour. The formula works well with any recipe that calls for white flour. Use about six cups of well-stirred and sifted mix in the recipe below.

Measure three cups of warm water (85°F) into a large bowl. Add two tablespoons of dry yeast granules (or two packets of yeast, or two squares of yeast) and two tablespoons of honey. Stir and allow the mixture to stand for five minutes.

By now the yeast mixture should be frothy. Stir into it one tablespoon of sea salt. Add half the flour mixture. Beat vigorously, using about seventy-five strokes by hand—or beat for two minutes if you are using an electric mixer.

Add two tablespoons of vegetable oil and the remainder of the flour mixture. Blend all of the ingredients thoroughly and turn the dough out onto a floured board. Have additional flour handy. Knead vigorously for about five minutes until the dough is smooth and elastic. Place it in an oiled bowl, oil the top of the dough lightly, and cover the bowl. Put it in a warm place (80°F-85°F) until it is nearly double in size. This will take about forty-five minutes.

Punch down the dough, fold over the edges, turn it upside down in the bowl, and let it rise another twenty minutes.

Turn the dough onto the board and divide it into three portions. Fold each one inward and form smooth, tight balls. Cover them with a clean cloth and allow them to rest ten minutes.

Shape into three loaves, or two loaves and a pan of rolls. Place in buttered tins (about 3½ by 7½ inches in size). Allow the dough to rise in the tins until it is doubled in bulk, about forty-five minutes. Bake in a preheated moderate oven (350°) for about fifty minutes. If the loaves begin to turn brown in fifteen to twenty minutes, reduce the temperature to 325°.

Remove the finished breads or rolls from the pans and cool them on racks. If desired, brush the tops with melted butter.

When you've grown accustomed to this recipe, you can add bran, beginning with one teaspoon per cup of flour and working your way upward.

This is an age of fast foods and quick indigestion, so here is a recipe for a quick bread that should *help,* rather than hinder, the digestive process.

Molasses Quick Bread

1½ cups of fine bran
1½ cups whole-wheat flour with 1 teaspoon
    wheat germ per cup
1½ cups buttermilk
1 teaspoon iodized salt
1 teaspoon baking soda
½ cup dark molasses
¼ cup raisins

Dissolve the baking soda in the molasses, stirring until doubled. Stir in bran, buttermilk, salt, raisins, and flour. Bake in an oiled loaf pan at 350° for about forty-five minutes.

Quick Whole-Wheat Wafers

1½ cups whole-wheat flour, sifted
½ cup bran
1 teaspoon iodized salt
½ cup heavy sweet cream, sour cream,
    milk, or yogurt

Blend flour, salt, and bran. Gradually work in the liquid. Toss dough onto a lightly floured pastry board and knead for about fifteen minutes. The dough should be stiff. Now roll until tissue thin, and cut into small strips or squares. Distribute on oiled cookie sheet, prick with fork, and bake until light brown—about eight to ten minutes—at 350°.

Sweetbreads

Gage needs on the basis of one and a half pounds of sweetbreads serving six. Do not presoak or precook sweetbreads if they are to be used immediately, but if they are not, precooking is mandatory, for, like all good foods, sweetbreads are highly perishable. To precook, simmer sweetbreads in water or stock to which you have added one teaspoon of salt and one tablespoon of lemon juice. After cooling, remove the loose membranes and refrigerate—and do use them as soon as possible.

Braised sweetbreads are simply prepared:

> 1½ pounds sweetbreads
> 3 tablespoons whole-wheat flour blended with 1 tablespoon bran
> 2 tablespoons sesame oil (or other preferred oil)
> Beef stock to cover (if you are stockless, use canned vegetable-beef soup, strained)

Wash sweetbreads, remove membrane, and dredge in flour-bran mixture. Heat oil, sauté sweetbreads briefly, pour stock over meat, and cover pan. Simmer gently for twenty minutes. Serves six.

Though the inexpensiveness of chicken is an illusion (the ratio of bones to meat is such that the net cost of chicken meat is about $1.50 per pound when the whole chicken sells at 59 cents per pound), I include a chicken recipe for those who are fond of chicken, and as an example of the way in which bran can be incorporated into everyday dishes.

Chicken en Casserole

1 large chicken, cut in six serving-size pieces
3 tablespoons oil
1 clove garlic
½ pound sliced mushrooms
1½ cups sweet cider
1 dozen small white onions stuck with cloves
2 diced carrots
1 stalk chopped celery, including leafy top
¼ cup bran and ¼ cup soy grits soaked in
    ½ cup stock (beef-vegetable or vegetable)
1 bay leaf
¼ teaspoon each of thyme, tarragon, basil
3 tablespoons minced parsley
1 teaspoon iodized salt
3 tablespoons brewer's yeast (not for leavening—do not use baker's yeast)
1 tablespoon soy flour

Rub chicken with garlic and sauté in hot oil. After removing chicken, sauté mushrooms in the same oil. Arrange mushrooms and chicken at the bottom of a casserole dish. Blend all other ingredients, pour over chicken and mushrooms, cover casserole, and bake at 350° for about one hour or until chicken is tender. Serves six.

Here's a good example of a high-fiber dessert that isn't laden with sugar.

Apple Brown Betty

1 cup whole-wheat bread crumbs or graham
    cracker crumbs, plus 1 cup bran
½ cup wheat germ
½ cup margarine, melted
2½ cups apples, cut up, with peels left on
½ cup seedless raisins
2 tablespoons honey
⅓ cup brown sugar
¾ teaspoon cinnamon
¼ teaspoon nutmeg
⅛ teaspoon cloves
½ teaspoon iodized salt
1 tablespoon lemon juice in ¼ cup water

Combine crumbs, wheat germ, bran, and melted butter. Cover bottom of a lightly greased baking dish with about one third of t' is mixture. In a bowl, sprinkle apples and raisins with honey and toss lightly to distribute evenly. In another bowl, combine sugar with spices and salt and mix well.

Put half the honeyed apple-raisin mixture over the crumbs in the baking dish and sprinkle with half the sugar-spice mixture and half the lemon water. Cover with another layer (one third) of the crumb mixture, then add the rest of the apples. Sprinkle with the remaining sugar-spice mixture and lemon water. Top with the final third of the crumbs.

Cover baking dish and bake at 350° for thirty-five minutes. Remove cover, increase heat of oven to 400°, and brown for ten to fifteen minutes. Serve hot with whipped cream, sour cream, or plain yogurt with vanilla. Serves four to six.

Snacks seem an unlikely vehicle for bran, but a little imagination produces one like this.

Stuffed Egg Snack

    3 eggs
    1 ounce margarine, melted
    ⅛ teaspoon iodized salt
    Very small pinch pepper
    ⅛ teaspoon prepared mustard
    2 tablespoons bran
    ½ teaspoon onion
    About 1/6 cup of flaked tuna, chopped
        shrimp, or crab meat

Hardcook eggs, and when they are cool, peel and cut in half lengthwise. Remove yolks and set whites aside. Mash yolks thoroughly—until crumbly—and then add margarine and all the other ingredients. Mix well—until smooth. Refill hollows in whites and garnish with olives.

Here's a good one-dish meal.

High-Protein-and-Vitamin Bake

1 pound pork sausage meat (choose a brand
   that does not contain BHT or BH/)
4 cups milk
½ cup skim-milk solids
½ cup undegerminated yellow cornmeal
½ cup wheat germ
¼ cup bran
1 teaspoon iodized salt
1 cup grated yellow cheese
4 eggs, separated

Shape sausage meat into flat patties and brown slowly (without adding fat) about five minutes to each side. Remove and drain on paper towels. Combine liquid and powdered milk thoroughly (you might use your blender at a slow speed), and scald three cups of the mixture. Slowly stir in cornmeal, wheat germ, bran, salt, and grated cheese. Mix well and cook over low heat, stirring continuously, until cheese melts and mixture thickens—about five minutes. Remove from heat and stir in remaining cup of (cold) milk. Allow the mixture to cool.

Beat egg yolks until light and frothy and add them to cereal mixture, blending thoroughly. Beat egg whites until stiff and fold into mixture. Pour into lightly greased casserole dish, arrange partially cooked meat patties on top, and bake at 350° for forty minutes. Serves four to six.

This recipe offers an interesting new flavor and higher nutrition levels.

Peanut Butter Biscuits

2 cups whole-wheat or unbleached white flour
¾ teaspoon iodized salt (less if peanut
   butter is very salty)
¼ cup skim-milk solids
3 teaspoons double-acting baking powder
2 tablespoons bran
1 tablespoon brewer's yeast
4 tablespoons margarine
4 tablespoons peanut butter
1 cup milk
1 tablespoon dark molasses or honey

Mix dry ingredients. Cream margarine with peanut butter, and cut this blend into the dry ingredients with a pastry blender or two knives. Add milk and molasses (or honey) and mix briskly with fork. Drop mixture by the spoonful onto a greased cookie sheet or into greased muffin tins and bake at 450° for fifteen minutes. Makes twelve to fifteen biscuits.

Betty is the woman who had the courage to cook and bake for her nutritionist husband. This recipe combines excellent nutrition and flavor.

Betty's Cookies

1 cup margarine
3 tablespoons sugar
1 egg or 2 yolks
2 level teaspoons baking powder
1 teaspoon vanilla
½ cup soybean flour
2 cups unbleached white flour
1½ teaspoons wheat germ
1 tablespoon bran
3 tablespoons skim-milk solids

Cream margarine and sugar. Add egg or yolks and blend well; then add remaining ingredients one at a time, blending thoroughly. Drop by teaspoonfuls onto greased cookie sheets and bake at 375° for fifteen minutes. Makes about four dozen.

Note: The content of soy flour, wheat germ, skim milk solids, and bran in these cookies can be raised until the end result has a protein level close to that of meat. Try the recipe in its present form. Next time, increase the quantity of one of these special ingredients a little. You'll eventually find the limits to the amounts of soy flour, wheat germ, skim-milk solids, and bran you can add and still have these cookies please your family.

From the South comes a good recipe for steak.

Southern Country-Fried Steak

Cube steak (or round steak) cut for individual
    servings
2 or 3 small onions
¾ cup unbleached flour mixed with ½ cup
    bran
Salt and pepper to taste

Salt and pepper steaks and dredge in flour. Brown quickly in a bit of hot fat. Remove steaks and brown the remaining flour in the steak drippings. Season to taste, and add chopped onions and enough water or milk to make a thick gravy. Place the steaks in the gravy, cover, and bake for two hours at 300°. Serve steaks without gravy if you wish.

Finally, for stuffing for turkey and other fowl you can use one and a half cups of bran to each eight cups of small, whole-grain bread cubes, plus your usual ingredients and seasonings. A teaspoonful of wheat germ may be added to each cup of the bran-bread mix.

You have already been told that coarse bran is more effective in aiding the physiological processes than fine bran is, but that some people tolerate fine bran better. When adding bran to recipes, you must keep in mind which type you're using, for their effects on baked recipes are different. In general, with coarse bran you'll need three tablespoons of extra liquid for each cup of bran. The liquid may be water or vegetable oil. With fine bran, you'll usually need to add only an extra tablespoon or so of oil or liquid per cup of bran. Where you do not wish to add extra vegetable oil or fluid to a recipe, an extra egg will often balance the effect of the added bran.

These specifications are aimed at helping you achieve an acceptable texture in a baked recipe, and, naturally, only experienc? will tell you what proportions of liquid shortening or other liquids will create the texture you and your family desire in your baked foods. You will therefore have to do some experimenting at first, but this bit of extra trouble will be well worth your while.

22. A Parting Word to the Nutritionally Wise

If you really want to profit by your high-fiber diet, don't lean on the use of added bran and wheat germ alone. Emphasize the foods in which fiber is retained. Avoid white flour, sugar of *any* color, white rice, degerminated cornmeal, processed rye, and processed buckwheat. (Few people realize that commercial rye bread is like white bread, and that commercial pumpernickel is a fermented rye bread artificially darkened with caramel color—burned sugar. They've all lost most of their fiber and all of their whole grain.)

In general, keep away from foods into which man's hands, techniques, and machines have intruded. Nobody can do anything to an egg except by failing to refrigerate it—or by marketing a substitute for it, which really is an insult both to the hen and to man! "Imitation," "synthetic," "equivalent," "processed"—these are emotionally charged words to the objective nutritionist.

If you're going to make a determined effort to

increase your intake of whole grain, to avoid fiber-free foods, and to cut down on your sugar consumption, you may wonder whether it is advisable to use *extra* bran and wheat germ. It is, for many good reasons. You have already learned that "whole grain" doesn't mean 100 per cent retention of fiber; it is unavoidable that some of it will be lost in the milling process. You will still be consuming sugar in significant amounts, because it is almost impossible to avoid. Finally—and this is probably the most significant factor of all in creating your need for supplementary bran and wheat germ—your capacity for eating whole grains is limited by your personal calorie ceiling. In this mechanized civilization, that capacity is probably low.

So add your bran, your wheat germ, and your yogurt to your diet. If your food selections in the past have been what I think they were (which brings up the whole question of how you survived to read this book), you should also start using B-complex and multiple vitamin-and-mineral supplements. It takes more than a good diet to compensate for years of inadequate nutrition.

And don't give me the argument that you feel fine. That puts you in the same class as the man who steps off the roof of a high building and, en route to the sidewalk and oblivion, says: "I'm doing all right—so far." If you feel fine you can feel finer, and in case you want to learn more about good nutrition—for there *is* more to it than fiber, B complex, and minerals—I have appended a bibliography that lists some of the papers that document this book and some of the books you might add to your library. These will provide further help in feeding yourself for good health.

Bibliography

Antia, F.P., and Desai, H.G. 1974. "Letter: Colonic Diverticula and Dietary Fibre." *Lancet.* 1:814.

Antonis, A., and Bersohn, I. 1962. "The Influence of Diet on Faecal Lipids in South African White and Bantu Prisoners." *American Journal of Clinical Nutrition.* 11:143-55.

Arfdwidsson, S. 1964. "Pathogenesis of Multiple Diverticula of the Sigmoid Colon in Diverticular Disease." *Acta Chirurgica Scandinavica.* Supplement no. 342.

Aries, V., and Williams, R.F.O. 1970. "Bacteria and Aetiology of Cancer of the Large Bowel." *Lancet.* 1:95-99.

Aries, V., et al. 1969. "Bacteria and Aetiology of Large Bowel Cancer." *Gut.* 10:334-335.

Barker, T.C., McKenzie, J.C., and Yudkin, J. 1966. *Our Changing Fare.* London: MacGibbon and Kee.

Berman, P.M., and Kirsner, J.B. 1973. "Diverticular Disease of the Colon—the Possible Role of 'Roughage' in Both Food and Life." *American Journal of Digestive Diseases.* 18:506-07.

"Bran and Diverticular Disease." 1972. *British Medical Journal.* 2:408-09.

Bruce-Chwatt, L.J. 1972. "Effects of Dietary Fibre." *British Medical Journal.* 4:49-50.

BIBLIOGRAPHY

Buckley, R.M. 1967. "Patterns of Cancer at Ishaka Hospital in Uganda." *East African Medical Journal.* 44:165-68.

Burkitt, D.P. 1972. "Varicose Veins, Deep Vein Thrombosis, and Haemorrhoids: Epidemiology and Suggested Aetiology." *British Medical Journal* 2:556-61.

————. 1973. "Some Diseases Characteristic of Modern Western Civilization." *British Medical Journal.* 1:274-78.

Burkitt, D.P., and James, P.A. 1973. "Low-Residue Diets and Hiatus Hernia." *Lancet.* 1:128-30.

Burkitt, D.P., Walker, A.R., and Painter, N.S. 1972. "Effect of Dietary Fibre on Stools and Transit-Times and Its Role in the Causation of Disease." *Lancet.* 2:1408-12.

Carlson, A.J., and Hoezel, F. 1949. "Relation of Diet to Diverticulosis of the Colon in Rats." *Gastroenterology.* 12:108-15.

Cowgill, G.R., and Anderson, W.E. 1932. "Laxative Effects of Wheat Bran and Washed Bran in Healthy Men. A Comparative Study." *Journal of the American Medical Association.* 98:1866-75.

Davies, J.N.P., Knowelden, J., and Wilson, B.A. 1965. "Incidence Rates of Cancer in Kyandondo County, Uganda, 1954-60." *Journal of the National Cancer Institute.* 35:789-821.

"Dietary Management of Diverticular Disease." 1973. *Journal of the American Dietetic Association.* 63:527-30.

Dimock, E.M. 1937. "The Prevention of Constipation." *British Medical Journal.* 2:906-09.

"Diverticular Disease of the Colon and Constipation

and Their Relationship to Our Diet." 1972. *Nursing Times*. 68:564-65.

"Diverticular Disease of the Colon and Constipation. 3. High-Fibre Diet with Added Bran." 1972. *Nursing Times*. 68:620-21.

Dodds, C., Fisher, N., Greenwood, C.T., and Hutchinson, J.B. 1972. "Effects of Dietary Fibre." *British Medical Journal*. 3:472-73.

Eastwood, M.A., and Girdwood, R.H. 1968. "Lignin: A Bile Salt Sequestrating Agent." *Lancet*. 2:1170-72.

Eastwood, M.A., Hamilton, T., Kirkpatrick, J. R., and Mitchell, W.D. 1973. "The Effects of Dietary Supplements of Wheat Bran and Cellulose on Faeces." *Proceedings of the Nutrition Society*. 32:22A.

Edington, G.M. 1956. "Malignant Disease in the Gold Coast." *British Journal of Cancer*. 10:595-608.

"The Effects of Dietary Supplements of Wheat Bran and Cellulose upon Bowel Function." 1972. *British Journal of Surgery*. 59:910.

Gustafsson, B.E., and Norman, A. 1969. "Influence of the Diet on the Turnover of Bile Acids in Germ-Free and Conventional Rats." *British Journal of Nutrition*. 23:429-42.

Harvey, R.F., Pomare, E.W., and Heaton, K.W. 1973. "Effects of Increased Dietary Fibre on Intestinal Transit." *Lancet*. 1:1278-80.

Heaton, K.W. 1973. "Food Fibre as an Obstacle to Energy Intake." *Lancet*. 2:1418-21.

———. 1974. "Letter: Dietary Fibre and Energy Intake." *Lancet*. 1:368-69.

BIBLIOGRAPHY

Hill, M.J., et al. 1971. "Bacteria and Aetiology of Cancer of the Large Bowel." *Lancet*. 1:95-99.

Hinton, J.M., Lennard-Jones, J.E., and Young, A.C. 1969. "A New Method for Studying Gut Transit Times Using Radio-Opaque Markers." *Journal of the British Society of Gastroenterology*. 10:842.

Hoffman, K. 1964. "Studies on the Composition of Fecal Flora During a Long-Term Nutrition Experiment with a High-Carbohydrate, High-Fat, and High-Protein Diet." *Zentralblatt für Bakteriologie*. 192:500-08.

Hoppert, C.A., and Clark, A.J. 1945. "Digestibility and Effect on Laxation of Crude Fiber and Cellulose in Certain Common Foods." *Journal of the American Dietetic Association*. 2:157-60.

Irving, D., and Drasar, B.S. 1973. "Fibre and Cancer of the Colon." *British Journal of Cancer*. 28:462-63.

Jones, C.R. 1958. "The Essentials of the Flour-Milling Process." *Proceedings of the Nutrition Society*. 17:7-15.

Kim, E.H. 1964. "Hiatus Hernia and Diverticulum of the Colon. Their Low Incidence in Korea." *New England Journal of Medicine*. 106:555-58.

Kramer, P. 1964. "The Meaning of High- and Low-Residue Diets." *Gastroenterology*. 47:649-52.

Lacassagne, A., Buu-Hoi, N.P., and Zajdela, F. 1961. "Carcinogenic Activity of Apcholic Acid." *Nature*. 190:1007-08.

Latto, C., Wilkinson, R.W., and Gilmore, O.J.A. 1973. "Diverticular Disease and Varicose Veins." *Lancet*. 1:1089-90.

"Laxatives and Dietary Fiber." 1973. *Medical Letter on Drugs and Therapeutics.* 15:98-100.

"Letter: Bile-Salt Patterns in Nigerians on a High-Fibre Diet." 1974. *Lancet.* 1:1002.

"Letter: Effect of Bran on Bowel Functions." 1973. *British Medical Journal.* 4:614.

Linsell, C.A. 1967. "Cancer Incidence in Kenya, 1957-64." *British Journal of Cancer.* 21:465-73.

Lynch, J.B., Hassan, A.M., and Omar, A. 1963. "Cancer in the Sudan." *Sudan Medical Journal.* 2:29-37.

McBee, R.H. 1970. "Metabolic Contributions of Cecal Flora." *American Journal of Clinical Nutrition.* 23:1514-18.

McCance, R.A., Prior, K.M., and Widdowson, E.M. 1953. "A Radiological Study of the Rate of Passage of Brown and White Bread Through the Digestive Tract of Man." *British Journal of Nutrition.* 7:98-104.

Morson, B.C., and Bussey, H.J.R. 1970. "Predisposing Causes of Intestinal Cancer." *Current Problems in Surgery.* February, pp. 1-46.

Mulligan, T.O. 1969. "The Pattern of Malignant Disease in Hesha, Western Nigeria." *British Journal of Cancer.* 24:1-10.

Oettle, A.G. 1964. "Cancer in Africa, Especially in Regions South of the Sahara." *Journal of the National Cancer Institute.* 33:383-439.

————. 1967. "Primary Neoplasms of the Alimentary Canal in Whites and Bantu of the Transvaal, 1949-53: A Histopathological Series." In *Tumors of the Alimentary Tract in Africans.*

National Cancer Institute monograph no. 25, pp. 97-110.

Painter, N.S., Almeida, A.Z., and Colebourne, K.W. 1972. "Unprocessed Bran in Treatment of Diverticular Disease of the Colon." *British Medical Journal.* 2:137-40.

Parks, T.G. 1973. "The Role of Dietary Fibre in the Prevention and Treatment of Diseases of the Colon." *Proceedings of the Royal Society of Medicine.* 66:681-83.

Parsons, D.S. 1973. "Dietary Fibre, Stool Output, and Transit-Time." *Lancet.* 1:152.

Payler, D.K. 1973. "Food Fibre and Bowel Behavior." *Lancet.* 1:1394.

Pomare, E.W., and Heaton, K.W. 1973. "Alteration of Bile-Salt Metabolism by Dietary Fibre (Bran)." *British Medical Journal.* 4:262-64.

"Possible Relationships Between Bowel Cancer and Dietary Habits." 1971. *Proceedings of the Royal Society of Medicine.* 64:964.

"Proceedings: The Effect of Bran on Transit Time, Bile-Acid Concentration, and Motility in Colonic Diverticular Disease." 1974. *British Journal of Surgery.* 61:323.

Robertson, J. 1972. "Changes in the Fibre Content of the British Diet." *Nature.* 238:290-92.

Schowengerdt, D.G., et al. 1969. "Diverticulosis, Diverticulitis and Diabetes." *Archives of Surgery.* 98:500-04.

Sealock, R.R., Basinski, D.H., and Murlin, J.R. 1941. "Apparent Digestibility of Carbohydrates, Fats, and Indigestible Residue in Whole-Wheat and White Breads." *Journal of Nutrition.* 22:589-96.

Sinclair, H. 1971. "Modern Diet and Degenerative Disease," in *Just Consequences*, ed. R. Waller. London: Charles Knight & Co., Ltd.

Stout, C., Morrow, J., Brandt, E.N., Jr., and Wolf, S. 1964. "Unusually Low Incidence of Death from Myocardial Infarction." *Journal of the American Medical Association*. 188:845-49.

Streicher, M.D., and Quirk, R.M. 1943. "Constipation: Clinical and Roentgenologic Evaluation of the Use of Bran." *American Journal of Digestive Diseases*. 10:179-81.

Walker, A.R.P. 1947. "The Effect of Recent Changes of Food Habits on Bowel Motility." *South African Medical Journal*. 21:590-96.

———. 1961. "Crude Fibre, Bowel Motility and Pattern of Diet." *South African Medical Journal*. 35:114-15.

———. 1971. "Diet, Bowel Motility, Faeces Composition and Colonic Cancer." *South African Medical Journal*. 45:377-79.

———. 1974. "Editorial: Dietary Fibre and the Pattern of Disease." *Annals of Internal Medicine*. 80:663-64.

Walker, A.R.P., Richardson, B.D., Walker, B.F., and Woolford, A. 1973. "Appendicitis, Fibre Intake and Bowel Behaviour in Ethnic Groups in South Africa." *Postgraduate Medical Journal*. 49:243-49.

Weisburger, J.H. 1973. "Chemical Carcinogenesis in the Gastrointestinal Tract." In *Seventh National Cancer Conference Proceedings*. Philadelphia: J.B. Lippincott Co.

Westhuizen, J. van der, Mbizvo, M., and Jones,

J.I. 1972. "Letter: Unrefined Carbohydrate and Glucose Tolerance." *Lancet.* 2:719.

Wozasek, O., and Steigmann, F. 1942. "Studies on Colon Irritation. III. Bulk of Faeces." *American Journal of Digestive Diseases.* 9:423-25.

Wynden, E.L., and Shigematsu, T. 1967. "Environmental Factors of Cancer of the Colon and Rectum." *Cancer.* 20:1520-61.

Books for a Nutritious Library

My library represents a forty-year accumulation of papers, abstracts, books, journals, and microfilm on nutrition. Many of them announced startling discoveries in the field, or monopolized on previously ignored truths. And many of them are now of historical significance only—their "truths" have been revealed as errors or (and this may be worse) half-truths.

Surviving the attrition of the decades are certain books that I think are of lasting value, and I am in no way deterred by false modesty in listing a few of my own among them. If I couldn't get another copy, I would never give away or lend:

Look Younger, Feel Healthier, by Carlton Fredericks. Grosset and Dunlap, New York.

Low Blood Sugar and You, by Carlton Fredericks. Grosset and Dunlap, New York.

Nutrition and Physical Degeneration, by Dr. Weston Price. Price-Pottenger Foundation, Los Angeles.

Nutrition in a Nutshell, by Dr. Roger J. Williams. Dolphin Handbooks, New York.

BOOKS FOR A NUTRITIOUS LIBRARY

PsychoNutrition, by Carlton Fredericks. Grosset and Dunlap, New York.

The Saccharine Disease, by T. L. Cleave, M.D. Keats Publishing, New Canaan, Connecticut.

Soil, Grass, and Cancer, by André Voison. Crosby Lockwood & Son, Ltd., London.

Sweet and Dangerous, by Dr. John Yudkin. Bantam Books, New York.

After you have read these, you will surely change your diet for the better—and then your health will change for the better too!

—CARLTON FREDERICKS

Index

About the Author

Carlton Fredericks, B.A., M.A., Ph.D., is a public-health educator who has specialized in nutrition education and research for thirty-five years. He has taught courses in the subject at City College of New York, Brooklyn College, New York University, Rockland (N.Y.) Community College, and New York Institute of Technology, and has also taught as a visiting clinician in the graduate continuing-education program of the School of Dentistry, University of Southern California. At present, Dr. Fredericks is a visiting professor of education at the College of Education, Fairleigh Dickinson University, where he teaches undergraduate and graduate courses in nutrition. He also teaches at Mercy College in Dobbs Ferry, N.Y., where he is a visiting professor of nutrition.

In 1975, Dr. Fredericks was elected president of the International Academy of Preventive Medicine and awarded an honorary life membership in the Academy of Medical Preventics. He is also a founding fellow of the International College of Applied Nutrition and an associate member of the Academy of Orthomolecular Psychiatry.

Dr. Fredericks is the author of numerous books on nutrition, among which are several best sellers. These include *Nutrition, Your Key to Good Health,*

ABOUT THE AUTHOR

Look Younger, Feel Healthier, and *Low Blood Sugar and You,* a pioneering text widely used as a reference book by both profe~sionals and the public. His newest release is *PsychoNutrition,* a work dedicated to orthomolecular psychiatry.